Breast or Bottle?

Studies in Rhetoric/Communication
Thomas W. Benson, Series Editor

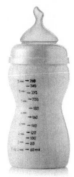

Breast or Bottle?

Contemporary Controversies in Infant Feeding Policy and Practice

Amy Koerber

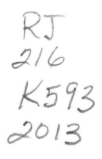
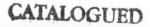

The University of South Carolina Press

© 2013 University of South Carolina

Published by the University of South Carolina Press
Columbia, South Carolina 29208

www.sc.edu/uscpress

Manufactured in the United States of America

22 21 20 19 18 17 16 15 14 13   10 9 8 7 6 5 4 3 2 1

Library of Congress Cataloging-in-Publication Data

Koerber, Amy (Amy Lunn)
Breast or bottle? : contemporary controversies in infant-feeding policy
and practice / Amy Koerber.
pages cm.—(Studies in rhetoric/communication)
Includes bibliographical references and index.
ISBN 978-1-61117-241-6 (pbk. : alk. paper)—ISBN 978-1-61117-246-1
(epub) 1. Infants—Nutrition. 2. Breastfeeding. 3. Bottle feeding.
I. Title.
RJ216.K593 2013
649'.33—DC23   2013007824

photograph of baby bottle © istockphoto.com/Ljupco

For Anne Berger, in loving memory

SOCRATES: That is just what surprises me, Gorgias, and has made me ask you all this time what in the world the power of rhetoric can be. For, viewed in this light, its greatness comes over me as something supernatural.

GORGIAS: Ah yes, if you knew all, Socrates,—how it comprises in itself practically all powers at once! And I will tell you a striking proof of this: many and many a time have I gone with my brother or other doctors to visit one of their patients, and found him unwilling either to take medicine or submit to the surgeon's knife or cautery; and when the doctor failed to persuade him I succeeded, by no other art than that of rhetoric. . . . So great, so strange, is the power of this art.

PLATO, *Gorgias*, circa 386 B.C.E.

Contents

6

Feminism, Rhetoric, and Breastfeeding
Some Concluding Remarks   *130*

Series Editor's Preface

Amy Koerber writes that scientific evidence in recent decades strongly supports the value of infant breastfeeding because of its profound benefits in strengthening the human immune system. This support has been a major shift in the public framing of scientific thinking. And yet, she argues in *Breast or Bottle? Contemporary Controversies in Infant Feeding Policy and Practice*, the shift in scientific thinking itself and the larger social discussion of infant-feeding practices, was preceded and continues to be strongly influenced by a variety of rhetorical currents. Promotion of and resistance to breastfeeding, with entailments in feminist and scientific discourse, have a complex history, a history complicated by the commercial interest in bottle feeding. Koerber explores the rhetoric of these discourses as they appear in research articles, advice literature, and policy documents. A rich series of interviews, conducted over a period of ten years with mothers, consultants, advocates, and medical authorities, brings context and perspective to this textual analysis.

Professor Koerber shows how, even when, midcentury medical experts supported breastfeeding as a foundation, they often understood breastfeeding as a model for the development of a commercially manufactured, testable, controllable, bottled baby milk based on cow's milk, with the guiding assumption that nutrition science could produce a commercial milk equivalent to, or even superior to, human milk. By the late twentieth century, it became more common to argue for the unique benefits of human milk for infant feeding. Earlier, breastfeeding had been the foundation; in an emerging formulation, breastfeeding was advocated as the norm, with the consequence of introducing a polarizing debate centering on the possible risks of bottle feeding. Professor Koerber's study of the commonplaces invoked by advocates shows how strongly medical and scientific discourse have been flavored by larger cultural shifts and how advocates and mothers themselves frame their views as invocations of science. At the same time, feminist advocates and the society at large have not come to terms with what it would mean for twenty-first century American mothers to breastfeed their babies. The rhetorical history offered in *Breast or Bottle?* is an important contribution to our understanding of the role of science in public-policy rhetoric and of the surprising turns in just half a century in the way we talk about a fundamental human practice. Koerber's study makes visible the structures of this talk and calls for a renewed feminist discourse on breastfeeding.

Acknowledgments

Although it seems like a long time ago, acknowledgments for this project extend all the way back to my dissertation at the University of Minnesota. In writing the dissertation, I benefited greatly from mentoring and writing guidance from my advisor Mary Lay Schuster and from committee members Laura Gurak, Arthur Walzer, and Karlyn Kohrs Campbell. These are the people who taught me how to think like a rhetorician, a habit I've never been able to break.

Since joining the faculty at Texas Tech University in 2002, I have received generous financial support from the College of Arts and Sciences, the EXPORT Center for Rural Health, and the School of Nursing. Such support has paid for graduate research assistants, travel to Elk Grove, Illinois, to conduct archival research at the American Academy of Pediatrics (AAP) headquarters, technology needs, and a faculty development leave in Fall 2009 that allowed me to finish an early version of this manuscript. I have enjoyed many conversations with Texas Tech colleagues over the years and am especially grateful for publishing advice offered by Sam Dragga and mentoring from Laura Beard. I have discussed infant feeding at great length with Linda Brice and Elizabeth Tombs from the Texas Tech University Health Sciences Center Anita Thigpen Perry School of Nursing and enjoyed having them as co-investigators in the focus-group research that informs some of this book's arguments. I have received excellent research assistance at various stages from Tamra Cumbie, Ryan Hoover, and Lonie McMichael. Although there are too many to name each one individually, I am also grateful to all the students who have enrolled in my graduate seminar in medical rhetoric over the years; the discussions in this class have contributed more to this book than these students will ever know.

I am thankful to the many women and men who participated in interview and focus-group research over the years. Although these participants must remain anonymous, I hope I have adequately and fairly recounted the stories they have told and that the resulting knowledge will benefit others who might encounter situations similar to those that the research participants have so generously shared. I am also thankful to John Zwicky, archivist at the American

Academy of Pediatrics History Center, and the staff at the Bakwin Library at AAP headquarters. These individuals also made it possible for me to visit the AAP headquarters and conduct archival research that has added important historical detail to many of the arguments presented in this book.

Since the moment I first considered submitting a proposal to University of South Carolina Press, I have received wonderful support and guidance from Jim Denton, acquisitions editor. Everyone at the press has been delightful to work with, and I have appreciated their clear guidance and responsiveness at every step of the way. I also received valuable feedback from Bernice L. Hausman and another, anonymous manuscript reviewer. I am also thankful to Dr. Lawrence Gartner, who participated in two telephone interviews and offered critical feedback on an early version of the manuscript. For scholarly inspiration and support, I am especially grateful to Judy Segal, who encouraged me at a time when I really needed it and whose work continues to remind me how great are the powers of rhetoric.

I am grateful to my father, who taught me the value of a good argument and was one of the first to give me critical feedback on my writing. My mother and father paid for my college education and enabled me to follow my dreams, even when those dreams did not seem so practical. I hope I can do the same for my own children.

I would have never thought of this project if not for long conversations I had with my mother, Gayle Backes, and her mother, Anne Berger, about the not-so-distant history of infant-feeding practices and recommendations in the United States. Both women breastfed their babies before it was sanctioned by medical experts and in times when it was not fashionable to do so. When my grandmother nursed her babies in the 1940s, she had to hide the practice from her pediatrician. She passed away early in 2011, and this book is dedicated to her loving memory.

And, finally, I have discovered along the way that writing books is a lot like raising children: both jobs require a lot more work than you envision at the outset, but they are also more rewarding than anyone could ever imagine. Most important, though, is that both jobs can be successful only when they are collective endeavors. In my case, I could not have completed this project without my husband and best friend, Brian Still. Brian made it just as possible to write when I had one tiny infant as it is now with a noisy but happy bunch that includes thirteen-year-old Jack, eight-year-old Olivia, and four-year-old Abraham.

Portions of chapter 2 and chapter 5 have been previously published as articles. An earlier version of chapter 2 was published as "From 'Wives' Tales and Folklore' to Scientific Fact: Rhetorics of Breastfeeding and Immunity, 1950–1997," in the *Journal of Medical Humanities* 27.3 (Fall 2006): 151–66. It is reprinted here with permission from Springer Publishing Company. An earlier version of chapter 5 was published as "Rhetorical Agency, Resistance, and the Disciplinary Rhetorics of Breastfeeding," in *Technical Communication Quarterly* 15.1 (January 2006): 87–101. It is reprinted here with permission from Taylor & Francis Ltd, http://www.tandf.co.uk/journals.

The image "Breastfeeding: Baby's First Immunization" is used with permission of the American Academy of Pediatrics, http://www2.aap.org/breastfeeding/curriculum/documents/pdf/BFIZPoster.pdf, copyright American Academy of Pediatrics, 2007.

Introduction

Just a few decades ago, the notion that human milk contains immune-protective qualities was routinely dismissed by medical experts, even referred to as the stuff of "wives' tales and folklore."[1] Now the American Academy of Family Physicians states in a position paper that "not breastfeeding is associated with increased risks of common conditions including acute otitis media, gastroenteritis, atopic dermatitis, and life-threatening conditions including severe lower respiratory infections, necrotizing enterocolitis, and sudden infant death syndrome."[2] In conjunction with this shift regarding what counts as scientific truth about human milk's immune-protective qualities, during the last few decades we have seen a profound shift in some of the medical recommendations on infant feeding and a less tangible, but equally profound, shift in popular understandings of what it means to make an infant-feeding choice. Whereas the phrase *breast or bottle* might have once implied a choice between two relative equals, each with its own benefits and drawbacks, we increasingly live in a world in which human milk is portrayed as possessing unique qualities that might be emulated but will never be replicated in an artificial substitute. As the American Academy of Pediatrics (AAP) proclaims in its current policy statement on infant feeding, breastfeeding is "the reference or normative model against which all alternative feeding methods must be measured with regard to growth, health, development, and all other short- and long-term outcomes."[3]

It is tempting to view this recent shift in beliefs as a typical example of science doing what it is supposed to do—increasing our knowledge and understanding of phenomena in the natural world—and medicine doing what it is supposed to do—changing its practices and recommendations in response

1

to relevant scientific advances. I argue in this book, however, that such a progress-based interpretation leads to an incomplete understanding of the recent shift in scientific facts and medical recommendations with regard to infant feeding.

Of course, the amount of epidemiologic evidence that demonstrates human milk's health benefits has increased in recent years, and so has the amount of evidence that helps us scientifically understand the mechanisms that lead to these benefits. But the story of why these forms of evidence have increased so dramatically in the last few decades is not just a story of new scientific discoveries. Rather, it is a story about individuals, coalitions, and organizational entities who have engaged in relentless rhetorical efforts to improve our scientific explanations and cultural appreciation of human milk, lactation, and breastfeeding in the context of a decades-long historical tendency to devalue and denigrate these uniquely female capabilities of the human body. Experts and advocates arguing in favor of human milk have gained important rhetorical ground since the 1970s when a shift in the dominant metaphor for the human immune system enabled medical researchers to start seeing human milk as part of this gender-neutral system instead of just an element of female reproduction. Prior to this important change in the rhetorical framework of the breast–bottle debate, researchers in pediatrics, immunology, and other medical specialties viewed human milk and breastfeeding as uniquely female capacities, and they were quite successful in accumulating evidence to argue against the idea that human milk provides any health benefits that cannot be duplicated in formula. When we acknowledge these important rhetorical shifts, events, and initiatives, it becomes clear that science should be understood as an important and ever-shifting frame for the breast–bottle controversy, but not as its final arbiter.

If we take seriously the excerpt from Plato's dialogue *Gorgias* that appears as an epigraph to this book, then considering the rhetorical aspects of a phenomenon such as infant feeding is crucial to developing a complete understanding of it. In fact, if we believe Plato's dialogue, those rhetorical dimensions might be even more important than the strictly scientific or medical dimensions at times and, in any case, hard to separate from them. Rhetoric has been defined, most simply and elegantly, as the capacity "to see the available means of persuasion in each case."[4] But the simplicity of this definition belies its true power. As suggested by Gorgias' reply to Socrates' question, Western culture has long acknowledged the mystical force of rhetoric and has even treated it as supernatural. As has been shown to be the case for the language that is used to talk about fertility, migraines, depression, and a variety of other health-related topics, the rhetoric used to promote breastfeeding at a given time and cultural moment is significant,[5] and it deserves close attention, because such language not only reflects a presumably preexisting reality but also actually plays a part in shaping that reality. Thus, it matters whether mothers are told simply that "breast is best" or whether they are hearing one of the current variations on this phrase: "Babies are born to be breastfed" and "Breast milk: Every ounce counts."[6]

The book's approach is best characterized as rhetorical history, or what Judy Segal has called "kairology." *Kairology* derives from the rhetorical principle of *kairos*, "the principle of contingency and fitness-to-situation."[7] A kairology, then, is "a study of historical moments [in medicine] as rhetorical opportunities."[8] In other words, the book's goals are to take a closer look at the multiple forms of rhetorical activity that have preceded the recent shift in scientific facts and medical recommendations with regard to infant feeding and to consider how these activities have altered the public space in which arguments about both breast- and bottle-feeding are made. In more specific terms, the rhetorical history offered in this book is motivated by the following questions:

- What kinds of changes need to come about for the potential health benefits of an activity such as breastfeeding to be described as "wives' tales and folklore" in one era but deemed so important that it is risky for an individual not to embrace such behavior just a few decades later?
- What kinds of persuasive activity have been necessary to articulate scientific and medical knowledge into new clinical practices and recommendations, and what are the obstacles to change in clinical practices?
- How does such a profound shift in scientific and medical beliefs shape the experiences of individuals who look to the medical establishment for guidance on a subject such as infant feeding?

Although these questions pertain to a specific era in the recent rhetorical history of infant feeding, the resulting analysis and conclusions, of course, pertain more broadly to major shifts in belief and practice—and the persuasive dimensions of such shifts—in other realms of health and medicine.

Feminism and Breastfeeding

The recent shift in the value that experts assign to breastfeeding has already received a considerable amount of scholarly attention, much of which has been informed by feminist perspectives. One important focal point of such research has been the National Breastfeeding Awareness Campaign (NBAC). Launched in 2004 by the United States Department of Health and Human Services, this campaign included television ads that used shocking depictions of a pregnant woman riding a mechanical bull and participating in a logrolling event while on-screen text asked mothers, "You wouldn't take risks before your baby's born. . . . Why start after?"[9] Feminist scholars have questioned the legitimacy of the scientific knowledge on which this breastfeeding campaign was based as well as the ethics of the campaign's rhetorical tactics. The most passionate and fully developed of such critiques is a recent book by Joan B. Wolf, who claims that the NBAC is based on faulty scientific evidence and is emblematic of a newly intensified public-health effort to mandate breastfeeding as part of an ideology of "total motherhood."[10]

Other feminist scholars share Wolf's concerns about some of the tactics being used to promote breastfeeding but do not share Wolf's skepticism about the science on which it is based. Rebecca Kukla is one such scholar. As Kukla says, "we have enough unequivocal data about the benefits of breastfeeding to make it clear that achieving and maintaining high rates of initiating and continuing breastfeeding should be important public health goals."[11] Instead, Kukla limits her criticism to the campaign's rhetorical strategy, which, she says, assumes that if women heard the message about human milk's health benefits packaged in the right way, they would start breastfeeding in larger numbers. As Kukla observes, there are likely many other factors influencing the breast-feeding decision and contributing to low rates, but the campaign does nothing to address these other factors.[12]

Because the rhetorical history presented in this book questions the prog-ress-based narrative of the recent shift in medical beliefs, it might seem to correspond with the findings of these feminist critical approaches. Ultimately, however, this book's argument departs from many of these feminist critiques and instead aligns more squarely with those feminist scholars who are call-ing for a discourse that explicitly supports breastfeeding. As one prominent example, Bernice L. Hausman takes issue with the way in which many femi-nist scholars approach what she calls the "scientific case for breastfeeding." Hausman accuses such scholars' analyses of dismissing the scientific case alto-gether or "emphasiz[ing] political concerns by repudiating scientific ones."[13] Rather than dismiss the recent explosion in scientific evidence for the benefits of breastfeeding, then, Hausman urges feminist scholars to use this explosion of medical attention as an occasion to insert a feminist voice into the multi-vocal, often antifeminist ideological battleground that currently constructs our culture's understanding of infant feeding. Specifically, Hausman argues, femi-nists should use the scientific case for breastfeeding that has emerged in recent decades as justification to fight for the kinds of pro-mothering workplaces and social reforms that feminists have been reluctant to fight for in the past.[14]

In hopes of working toward the goals that Hausman stipulates for feminist breastfeeding scholars, I argue in this book that a rhetorical perspective is cru-cial to developing a full understanding of the pro-breastfeeding messages that are circulating so widely in so many different channels today. If the exhortation to breastfeed is often delivered in a manner that seems overly strident, and if it seems like today's mothers are bombarded from all directions with the message that "breast is best," that is not just because of abstract forces or political entities that are trying to make today's mothers hyper-responsible for their infants' well-being. Rather, it is because today's pro-breastfeeding messages are being uttered in the context of a long anti-breastfeeding history. For those who have long advocated breastfeeding within this context, science-based messages that strongly articulate the unique health benefits of human milk and breastfeeding have been the only means of making effective arguments. If these science-based arguments have become increasingly intense in recent years, that is because the rhetorical situation has demanded such intensity.

By arguing that the recent intensification of beliefs in the health benefits of breastfeeding cannot be accurately understood apart from this larger context in which arguments about both breast and bottle are made and presented, then, I enter feminist discussions from a perspective that outwardly supports breastfeeding. When we take into account the larger cultural and rhetorical shifts that this book examines, today's pro-breastfeeding messages take on a different meaning. Although this different meaning emerges from an analysis that employs the techniques and disciplinary practices specific to rhetorical studies, it is a meaning of which scholars in feminist studies, science studies, public health, and related fields should be aware, regardless of whether such scholars are more inclined to agree with, to criticize, or to reject current breastfeeding messages. Viewed from the perspective of a history that has denigrated breastfeeding and human milk at every step of the way, the pro-breastfeeding exhortations that we hear today from medical and public-health authorities are shown to have complex layers of meaning in relation to our cultural understandings of motherhood and of women's bodies more generally. Furthermore, because the historical tendency to devalue human milk, breastfeeding, and lactation has been so profound and because the historical roots of this devaluation run so deep, the change that seems so dramatic when we look at the surface of official medical recommendations becomes less clearly defined when we look beyond that surface. In fact, the stories of mothers, breastfeeding advocates, and medical experts I have interviewed during the last decade indicate that historical tendencies to devalue breastfeeding and to hold human milk to a much higher standard than formula still persist in the contemporary United States. As a result, breastfeeding and human milk are still being treated as anything but normal in the United States today, and the apparently profound change in medical beliefs is actually far from complete. In fact, some sectors of the medical community and the public at large have been quicker than others to enact these changes. That is why today's mothers are hearing mixed messages, deeply conflicting ideas about how they should feed their infants, and it is also why many of the anti-breastfeeding messages still persist despite the current enthusiasm that appears on the surface of medical recommendations.

Acknowledging the multiple rhetorics that shape how both experts and nonexperts perceive infant feeding in the United States today and trying to gain some understanding of how these rhetorics interact has at least three distinct but interrelated benefits to readers of this book. First, it leads to a more complete understanding of the pro-breastfeeding messages that women are currently receiving. Yes, these messages are more intense than ever before. But that is not only because scientific evidence has accumulated over the years, nor is it only because, as some feminist scholars have asserted, the medical establishment wants to make mothers hyper-responsible for everything that happens to their children.[15] Calling both of these interpretations into question enables a perspective that situates current breastfeeding-promotion messages in relation to a history of weaker pro-breastfeeding stances that preceded it and illuminates the rhetorical activity that has been necessary to achieve and publicize current medical beliefs about infant feeding. Ultimately, I would hope, such an analysis might help today's parents engage in what Kimberly K. Emmons calls a "self-care" as they face the complex, and often emotionally intense, experiences of feeding and caring for infants in a society in which these aspects of life have become increasingly medicalized over the last century.[16] According to Emmons, a "rhetorical care of the self" builds on the increasingly intense reliance on self-doctoring and self-care that we are already experiencing in the twenty-first-century United States, but it demands "more complex responses" to the scientific and medical discourses that we so eagerly seek to help us understand not only infant feeding but a myriad of other health-related topics as well.[17]

Second, a rhetorical analysis acknowledges not only broad cultural forces such as "scientific progress" or "total motherhood ideology," which can sometimes seem impersonal or abstract, but also emphasizes the capacity of individual and organizational rhetors to intervene in scientific controversies and the responsibilities of various individuals to do so. Thus, a rhetorical analysis can help us identify the problematic interplay of infant-feeding messages as the root of mothers' current confusion and anxiety about infant feeding. If public health research has offered important insights in response to the question "Why would a woman not want to breastfeed, given all that is known about its health benefits?," we might say that many feminist scholars have turned this question around to ask "Why would a woman *want* to breastfeed, given the hidden uncertainties in current scientific knowledge and all the difficulties involved?"[18] A rhetorical study, in contrast to both of these other approaches, turns our attention away from narrowly circumscribed notions of individual choice and instead toward the larger environment in which medical-ized activities such as infant feeding occur. The layers of meaning that emerge through rhetorical analysis can be easily obscured in a catch phrase such as "breast or bottle," which reduces infant feeding to a seemingly simple matter of individual choice. Such an analysis can yield a more complex and nuanced understanding that will hopefully alter the tendency to blame individual moth-ers for either breastfeeding or not breastfeeding and will ultimately lead us to question whether health-related experiences such as infant feeding are even properly characterized in terms of choice. Along these lines, a rhetorical analy-sis helps us see the varying extents to which the changes in medical recommen-dations have impacted behaviors of different audiences and better understand the reasons for this uneven impact.

Third, a rhetorical analysis can enrich our understanding of the manner in which expert knowledge is produced and the channels through which indi-viduals in the public sphere receive and relate to such information. An impor-tant facet of such an analysis is the need not just to consider the rhetoric of physicians themselves but also to take a broader view of who is persuading and being persuaded by medical rhetoric. Thus, in this book, I look closely at the rhetorical activities of various stakeholders, including not only physicians and medical researchers but also policy makers, public-health authorities, market-ing professionals, health communicators, and mothers. This expanded view reveals a whole series of arguments, controversies, and other forms of rhetori-cal activity that can easily be obscured when we limit our understanding of scientific and medical change to a progress-based narrative.

Doing Rhetorical Analysis

The rhetorical history that this book offers is grounded in extensive research and analysis that I have conducted during the last decade, sometimes alone and sometimes as part of a research team. The ultimate goal of rhetorical analysis is, according to Judy Z. Segal, "a greater understanding of human action."[19] Along similar lines, Jack Selzer defines rhetorical analysis as "study-ing carefully some kind of symbolic action, often after the fact of its delivery and irrespective of whether it was actually directed to you or not, so that you might understand it better and appreciate its tactics."[20] In the broadest terms, these understandings of rhetorical analysis have informed my project from the beginning. To achieve the goals that scholars such as Segal and Selzer describe, I have read hundreds of relevant scientific texts, analyzed public-health messages, explored archives to uncover key policy documents, and interviewed various stakeholders in the breastfeeding controversy, including mothers themselves, all in attempt to illuminate the decades-long history of expert debate that has culminated in this apparent shift in what counts as fact in the context of scientific and medical practice. Specifically, I have examined a range of medical texts published from 1940 to the present, including research articles, advice literature, and policy documents. I have also examined meeting minutes, memos, and other technical documents that relate to the drafting of recent AAP policy statements on infant feeding. Many of the documents I have examined are publicly available in peer-reviewed journal articles or on websites. However, some of the documents were retrieved in March 2008 from the Pediatric Historical Archive of the AAP, an organizational archive located at the AAP Headquarters in Elk Grove, Illinois. These multiple forms and sources of textual analysis reflect the fact that, although this is a book about contemporary infant-feeding controversies, it also carefully considers how such controversies are shaped by past events, attitudes, and beliefs. Rather than looking at just the present situation, or at just the past, a rhetorical history stands apart from the other approaches that have been used to study infant feeding, because it requires us to view current controversies as they are unfolding in a situation that still contains important elements from the past.[21]

To contextualize these multiple forms of textual analysis, I have also conducted a series of interviews with various stakeholders in the breast–bottle debate. In the first phase of this research, I interviewed fifteen people involved in breastfeeding advocacy in order to understand both the exigency that led to the AAP's 1997 declaration of breastfeeding as the "reference or normative model" and the rhetorical effects of this declaration. The people interviewed in this first phase of research all considered themselves breastfeeding advocates, although they practiced their advocacy in different locations—some within the medical community and some beyond. Specifically, I interviewed two postpartum doulas, six La Leche League leaders, five lactation consultants, one woman involved in breastfeeding education and promotion through WIC (Women, Infants, and Children), and one woman who is both a La Leche League leader and a lactation consultant. This first phase of interviews was conducted from May to August 2000. All of these research participants identified their ethnicity as white.

The next phase of interviews was conducted in 2004. Participants in this phase included three breastfeeding advocates, women who worked with mothers in various capacities to support natural birth and breastfeeding in the Lubbock, Texas, area. I recruited these three women through a local organization that advocated natural childbirth and provided resources for mothers looking to have homebirths or unmedicated hospital births. I used this organization's listserv, along with snowball recruiting, to enlist nine participants who were mothers who had given birth in West Texas within the last ten years but were not actively involved in breastfeeding advocacy or support. Some of these women had breastfed their babies and some had not. Again, all participants identified their ethnicity as white.

The most recent research involving mothers was conducted when I served as part of an interdisciplinary team, which included two faculty members from the Texas Tech University Health Sciences Center Anita Thigpen Perry School of Nursing in addition to me. This phase of the research included a series of nine focus groups conducted from July to December 2008 in Lubbock, Texas. Participants were recruited from two different locations: Texas Tech University and a Lubbock community organization that provides support to under-privileged mothers. Women were eligible to participate in the study if they had given birth within the last three years or if they were currently expecting a child. A total of fifty-six participants enrolled in the study; forty-five of these were mothers who had given birth within the last three years or were currently expecting a child. The other eleven were friends, relatives, or partners who attended along with a mother. All mothers were invited to bring along one person, eighteen years of age or older, of their choosing. Based on responses to a demographic questionnaire that was filled out only by the mothers in the study, our sample included five participants who self-identified as Asian, two who self-identified as black or African American, eight who self-identified as Hispanic or Latino, three who self-identified as mixed race, and twenty-six who identified as white.

Finally, I conducted telephone interviews with Dr. Lawrence Gartner on November 13, 2000, and April 28, 2008. Gartner headed the AAP Work Group on Breastfeeding that authored the 1997 policy statement; this work group later became the AAP's Section on Breastfeeding that produced the statement published in 2005.[22]

Every interview and focus-group conversation was transcribed verbatim, sometimes by me and sometimes by a research assistant. I then analyzed these transcripts along with the other texts in a manner typical of rhetorical analysis. That is, I read and reread the texts, highlighting important themes and contin-ually seeking out new information that might call into question any tentative conclusions I might start to draw. This recursive approach has also informed my process of selecting texts and recruiting participants throughout the proj-ect. Because this is a qualitative study, the sample of texts I have analyzed and the sample of people I have interviewed over the years are not intended statistically to represent any particular phenomenon or demographic group. I have, however, adhered to widely accepted practices for effective sampling in qualitative research. In particular, each time I have progressed to a new phase of the research, I have purposely aimed to select texts and to recruit partici-pants who would force me to question the conclusions I was starting to draw about the previous phase of research. It has also been an overarching goal over the years to build a sample of texts that is increasingly rich and a pool of research participants that is increasingly diverse in terms of ethnicity and socioeconomic and other demographic factors. In qualitative research, these principles derive from techniques usually described as purposeful sampling or theoretical sampling. In purposeful sampling, the researcher "selects individuals and sites for study because they can purposefully inform an understanding of the research problem and central phenomenon in the study."[23] Theoretical sampling rests on similar principles, but it applies these principles in a way that is appropriate to a long-term multiphase study such as that which has led to this book. Specifically, theoretical sampling "begins with selecting and studying a homogeneous sample of individuals" and then attempts to build a sample that is increasingly heterogeneous as the study unfolds as a way "to confirm or disconfirm the conditions, both textual and intervening, under which the model holds."[24] Although there are subtle differences between these two sampling approaches, my research over the years has been influenced by both.

Some of the forms of rhetorical activity that are revealed in these chapters might seem tangentially, rather than directly, related to breastfeeding. For instance, in the field of immunology, metaphors that govern scientific understanding of the human immune system have dramatically changed in the last several decades, and these changes have led to popular and expert definitions of healthy bodies that are more favorable to arguments in support of breastfeeding's health benefits. Other forms of rhetorical activity have been more directly connected to breastfeeding advocates' strategic efforts. For instance, medical and public-health experts have engaged in arguments about the relationships between social and biological dimensions of mothering young children, pediatrics experts have engaged in rhetorical struggles to renegotiate their professional relationships with the formula industry, and our society as a whole has engaged in rhetorical struggles arising from questions about the human female body's ability to nourish an infant through lactation. Although they have occurred in different public spaces and at different times, these larger changes in cultural narratives and the more specific changes in scientific fact and medical practice collectively represent a shift in the contours of the set of alternatives that has come to be known in U.S. society through the catch phrase "breast or bottle." Through the rhetorical history that is presented in the next six chapters, I hope to enhance our understanding of this shift and also to suggest how such a rhetorical analysis can contribute more generally to our understanding of fundamental changes in what counts as truth in the context of contemporary Western medicine.

1

....

Infant Feeding and Rhetoric

An Overview

The recent intensification and proliferation of pro-breastfeeding messages in the United States can be traced to a highly publicized policy statement that the American Academy of Pediatrics (AAP) published in 1997. The statement urged women to breastfeed for at least the first year of the infant's life and stipulated that breastfeeding is "the reference or normative model against which all alternative feeding methods must be measured with regard to growth, health, development, and all other short- and long-term outcomes."[1] This statement represented a dramatic shift from the AAP's previous position on infant feeding and is perhaps the most significant rhetorical event in the recent history of infant-feeding controversies in the United States.

To justify the organization's dramatic shift in stance toward human milk and breastfeeding, the authors of the policy statement invoked a narrative of scientific progress. For instance, the statement begins with language that emphasizes the historical continuity of the organization's stance toward infant feeding. The opening paragraph declares that the AAP has "from its inception . . . been a staunch advocate of breastfeeding as the optimal form of nutrition for infants" and that "the activities, statements, and recommendations of the AAP have continuously promoted breastfeeding of infants as the foundation of good feeding practices."[2] The authors then proceed by attributing the academy's new stance to "considerable advances that have occurred in recent years in the scientific knowledge of the benefits of breastfeeding, in the mechanisms underlying these benefits, and in the practice of breastfeeding."[3] A 2005 revision of the earlier statement places a similar emphasis on scientific progress, claiming to reflect the "significant advances in science and clinical medicine" that had occurred since the 1997 statement.[4] Based on the language used in this narrative, we might surmise that the medical community has always supported breastfeeding but recent advances in understanding specific health benefits have intensified that support. Although the current recommendations differ from older recommendations, such language suggests, the difference is incremental and by no means revolutionary.[5]

A similar emphasis on scientific progress and newly discovered evidence was echoed in many of our focus-group participants' perceptions of current breastfeeding information.[6] In the words of Rebecca, who was expecting her first child at the time, "now there are more studies going on and more information out there about the benefits of breastfeeding." Another participant, Mary, had two young children when she participated in our focus group and had exclusively breastfed both children until the age of six months. Mary expressed a similar faith in the currently available scientific knowledge about breastfeeding: "That's just magical about breast milk. It's just so amazing. My friend went on a website, and she says there's, like, a jillion benefits. They're coming up constantly with all these benefits of breast milk."

Many participants echoed the policy statements' emphasis on novelty and scientific progress by stating that they felt fortunate to have access to more and better breastfeeding information than their own mothers had. As stated by Connie, a young mother who was expecting her first child at the time of focus-group participation, "I just get more information that my mom didn't know then. She, you know, I tell her and she's, like, 'Oh, I didn't know that.'" Andrea, who had breastfed her first child until the age of six months and her second child until the age of five months, also said that she had access to much better information than her own mother had: "I don't think she had near the information I have. I don't think there was any way she could have." And Nancy, who had exclusively breastfed her child until the age of five months, agreed: "I think for my mom, it wasn't the thing in her day either. And she didn't really care about it very much in the first place, but now there's so much education about the pros of it, that I think that a lot of women consider it."

Some focus-group participants were even more specific in their references to recent discoveries about the immune-system benefits of human milk. For instance, Mary went so far as to suggest that her husband's asthma could have been prevented if only his mother had had access to today's scientific knowledge: "So many things, and just all the time if you, you know, log on. And my husband, who was not breastfed . . . , he's asthmatic and they found that it prevents asthma. And that colostrum, they call it liquid gold and that actually coats their body and it helps their developing body and they just need all that. He was allergic to milk. He had all these things wrong with him. And I think breast milk would have prevented it."

These mothers' emphasis on novelty and advancement hints at the presence of a persuasive mechanism that Jeanne Fahnestock calls the "wonder appeal."[7] Such an appeal, quite typical in public representations of and responses to scientific knowledge, might suggest that the recent intensification of medical recommendations in support of breastfeeding has been the inevitable end result of a slow and steady climb toward a truer and better state of knowledge.

These mothers' comments, when considered alongside the narrative of scientific progress that is used to justify the medical establishment's increasing faith in human milk, raise some questions that serve as a useful starting place for a rhetorical investigation of infant feeding in the contemporary United States: How did we get to this moment? What does it mean to say that today's new mothers have more and better information about breastfeeding than their own mothers did? What kinds of breastfeeding facts are being established and communicated today, and why were these facts not available a generation ago?

We can begin to address such questions by sketching the contours of, as Judy Z. Segal says, a "rhetorically tilted medical history" of U.S. infant-feeding policy and practice as that history has unfolded from the mid–twentieth century to the present.[8] Attempting to "open up differences inside medicine and create better access to them" and to "interrogate that which is dismissed as 'what everybody knows,'" we can identify three distinctly different topoi, or rhetorical commonplaces, that have provided the basis for experts' arguments about breast- and bottle-feeding since the mid–twentieth century: the topos of breastfeeding as foundation in the mid–twentieth century, the topos of breastfeeding as the norm in the late twentieth century, and the topos of formula as risky in the early twenty-first century.[9]

Topoi have traditionally been understood as the commonplaces that serve as a conceptual inventory that speakers or writers at a particular historical moment can use to build their arguments. A particular topos can serve as effective material for an argument because it resonates as common sense with a given audience at a given place and time. However, to say that each of the historical moments examined in this chapter is defined by its own topos is not to say that other ideas have ceased to exist or to have any credibility at that moment. Rather, the notion of topos as rhetorical commonplace is meant to capture the predominant assumptions that shape what can be said and most readily accepted as true at a given historical moment—the argumentative material that is most easily available and, consequently, might ring true with a given audience at a given moment. The etymologic origins of *topos* link it to notions of physical place or space (as in *topography*, the study of place or, more specifically, physical features of a geographic location). So, in a quite literal manner, we might think of topos as a "conceptual place to which an arguer may mentally go to find arguments."[10] Taking a rhetorical approach to history, then, we might assume that a historical period is shaped by the kinds of commonplaces or stock material that are most readily available to the speakers and writers who are poised to make arguments on a particular subject in a particular place or time.

These connections to notions of place and physical location make the topos concept especially appropriate for conducting a rhetorical investigation of expert controversies on a subject such as infant feeding. The exact formulation of the concept has of course changed and evolved since Aristotle's time, but the current understanding is that topoi serve simultaneously as a means of decorum (that is, reinforcing conventional ideas) and as a means of invention (that is, making new ideas possible). In other words, as speakers and writers build arguments from these old materials, they put them together in new ways that can and often do result in new ideas. Thus, viewing scientific history through the lens of topoi entails an understanding of progress in which the kind of novelty that is so greatly emphasized in current infant-feeding rhetoric is seen as deeply rooted in old ideas. This makes the topoi concept especially well suited for reconsidering the narratives of scientific progress and the "wonder appeal" that are prevalent rhetorical features of current infant-feeding discourse. In so far as such arguments are built, at least in part, from conceptual inventories that are already available, we must temper our judgments about the actual novelty of ideas that are touted as the latest and greatest. In the case of infant feeding, each of the three topoi examined in this chapter has shaped what kind of knowledge can be produced and how that knowledge can be communicated to various audiences at a given historical moment. We might say such ideas have literally formed the topography of the rhetorical landscape that has surrounded infant-feeding controversies at each of these historical moments. Whereas subsequent chapters will look more closely at the rhetorical events that have led these three different commonplaces to emerge, change, and evolve, this chapter's aim is simply to introduce the three topoi as they have existed at different historical moments and to expose how each one has embodied its own unique set of assumptions for framing experts' arguments about breast- and bottle-feeding.

An important theme that emerges is a decades-long, ongoing shift in the ways that science has been invoked by advocates of both breastfeeding and bottle-feeding. In fact, each of the three topoi might be said to embody a different set of possibilities for the type of scientific evidence that can be used in making arguments about infant feeding and a different set of rules for how such evidence can be invoked. In the mid–twentieth century, the preponderance of scientific evidence worked in favor of the formula industry. Starting in the late twentieth century, and continuing into the present, the situation has changed in ways that seem to be making the available scientific evidence more favorable to breastfeeding advocates; that is, breastfeeding advocates have been able to use scientific evidence in ways that support an increasingly sharp distinction between human milk and formula. Even as this change has occurred, however, the pressure on those who advocate breastfeeding has continued to increase, so that breastfeeding advocates have been required to make increasingly strong arguments to support their claims that human milk is superior to artificial substitutes. Examining how each of these three topoi has coincided with a different set of possibilities for invoking scientific evidence in the breast–bottle debate offers additional texture to the narrative of gradual, incremental scientific progress that is apparent in official policy language and also in the remarks of focus-group participants.

Mid–Twentieth Century:
The Topos of Breastfeeding as Foundation

Because breastfeeding as foundation is the oldest of the three topoi, medical historians have already done much of the work necessary to understand how arguments about breast and bottle were made and received in the historical era defined by this topos. Such historians generally agree that the question of which feeding method was best for babies was subject to a great deal of uncertainty in early and mid-twentieth-century infant-feeding science.[11] As a result, although early and mid-twentieth-century medical experts might have outwardly expressed their support for breastfeeding, they construed breastfeeding as a model that formula producers should emulate as they sought to perfect their products and that mothers should emulate if they chose to bottle-feed with formula. In fact, as medical historians suggest, although official medical policy throughout the twentieth century has consistently expressed support of breastfeeding, by the 1940s most U.S. physicians had come to accept the idea that mass-produced artificial formulas derived from cow's milk could be a suitable, or even superior, substitute for human milk.[12] This belief created a rhetorical landscape in which breastfeeding and human milk often ended up being compared unfavorably to their artificial substitutes. Historian Rima D. Apple suggests that by the middle of the twentieth century many physicians were so enthusiastic about artificial formulas that they began to believe them superior to human milk, a belief that was reinforced by a number of studies that seemed to prove human milk unreliable because its vitamin contents were variable.[13] Thus, most of the mothers of the women who are the targets of today's medical discourse likely heard from their physicians that bottle-feeding with infant formula derived from cow's milk was an adequate, or superior, substitute for breastfeeding.[14]

The early twentieth century has received a great deal of attention from historians of medicine because this was the first time in medical history that a commercially produced, widely accessible alternative to human milk existed, and, in the early twentieth century, companies producing formulas were beginning to promote them to physicians and parents alike. Although, as Apple indicates, official medical discourse continued to espouse the view that breastfeeding was the ideal form of nourishment for babies, the increasing availability and quality of this commercial substitute around the turn of the century allowed them to assure their patients that, if they did not want to breastfeed or if they were unable to do so, bottle-feeding was an adequate substitute. At a time when faith in both medical science and artificial products was on the rise in the United States, this advice was readily accepted by new mothers eager to make the right choices about feeding their babies.[15]

Another factor that historians have noted is that in the mid twentieth century the formula industry stepped up its marketing efforts. Such efforts often targeted physicians and hospitals directly by providing them with free samples to distribute to their patients. The formula industry also became more heavily involved in funding medical research on infant feeding. A common feminist interpretation relates the early twentieth-century decline in breastfeeding to the increasing medical control over childbirth taking place at that time.[16] Indeed, bottle-feeding seemed more compatible with the medical model of childbirth and childrearing that was gaining increasing legitimacy in the early part of the twentieth century. If a woman bottle-fed, she could report to the physician exactly how much milk her baby consumed on a daily basis, and both mother and physician presumably could know the exact nutritional composition of what the baby was being fed. Giving the physician this kind of control over infant feeding was an important factor in the process through which pediatrics defined itself as a profession in the early part of the twentieth century.[17] By contrast, human milk and the practice of breastfeeding seemed more difficult to monitor. This imbalance created a situation in which breastfeeding and human milk came to be viewed as imperfect and unable to achieve the level of quality that could be achieved in artificial substitutes. As stated in one early twentieth-century medical publication that has been noted by medical historians, "it is easier to control cows than women."[18] Many medical studies at the time supported the belief that formula could be a superior substitute for human milk, particularly when administered as part of a physician-supervised feeding program.[19]

In rhetorical terms, emphasizing weight gain and protein levels appears to have enabled physicians to navigate the uncertainty that pervaded medical experts' discussions of infant feeding in the mid–twentieth century. Because there was so much uncertainty about the best feeding method, it appears that early twentieth-century physicians often looked to criteria that could be easily measured and monitored to make decisions about infant-feeding research and management. Apple's historical analysis suggests that early infant growth often was such a deciding factor. A central focus of physicians' concerns, according to Apple, was the observation that babies who were exclusively breastfed tended to lose weight in the first few days after birth, probably because mothers typically produce only colostrum, rather than fully developed milk, in these first few days. Physicians at the time believed colostrum contained little or no nourishment, and their fears were reinforced by the observation of initial weight loss in newborns who were exclusively breastfed.[20]

This historical literature hints at what I refer to as the topos of breastfeeding as foundation. But to understand how this topos functioned to enable certain kinds of arguments and preclude other kinds, we must look more closely at some examples of mid-twentieth-century medical texts. Such examples reinforce the recent AAP policy statements' assertions that the academy has throughout the twentieth century used language that consistently supports breastfeeding "as the optimal form of nutrition." However, when we look at the language used in mid-twentieth-century documents, it is clear that "breastfeeding as optimal" implies a set of conceptual resources for arguments about breast and bottle that is quite different from that implied by the organization's current stipulation that breastfeeding is the "normative model."

When we look closely at mid-twentieth-century medical texts, we can start to see what kinds of arguments are enabled by the topos of breastfeeding as foundation. In such texts medical professionals are urged to treat breastfeeding and human milk as foundational when they assist mothers in feeding their newborn infants or when they engage in research and development on new artificial substitutes for human milk. As a topos, the notion of breastfeeding as foundation seems to have functioned as a "conceptual framework that makes particular structures and lines of argument possible while foreclosing others."[21] For example, a section titled "The Mother's Role in the Feeding Program" in the published proceedings of a 1947 AAP panel discussion advises pediatricians that when a mother is bottle-feeding, she should try to imitate the physical actions involved in breastfeeding: "If the baby is to be bottle fed, the mother should at least cuddle him in her arms while he is taking his food in order to give him some physical semblance of the breast feeding."[22] Although this 1947 language acknowledges that breastfeeding is ideal, it also suggests a permissive, even encouraging, attitude toward artificial replacements: "If he seems to want it, she [the mother] may allow the baby to take sterile water or sugar solution from the bottle, as much as he seems eager for." More important, the document implies that an inadequate milk supply is a likely, perhaps the most likely, outcome for breastfeeding mothers, and it recommends feeding supplemental bottles of water or sugar water to prevent this situation: "Most pediatricians who are interested in breast feeding advise against the use of complemental feedings until the supply of breast milk has proved inadequate. It requires at least five to six days to make this diagnosis under ordinary conditions. Water or 5 percent solution of dextrose is usually given as desired, however. When this is done, dehydration fever or alarming loss of weight rarely occur."[23] Understanding the differences between breastfeeding as "optimal" and breastfeeding as "normative" is key to understanding the rhetorical situation of infant-feeding arguments that were made in the mid-twentieth-century United States. To treat these as two different rhetorical commonplaces is to consider how each formulation of the breast–bottle relationship has literally made possible some kinds of arguments in each historical era while precluding other kinds.

Shifting from advice literature to clinical research reports, we gain a more specific understanding of how the topos of breastfeeding as foundation facilitated arguments that devalued human milk and breastfeeding even while outwardly supporting them. For instance, in a 1948 study of premature infants the authors concluded that human milk is adequate for some, but not all, mothers and babies. Specifically, the article reports, "premature infants gain faster on half-skimmed milk than on human milk," and that, therefore, "the evidence is against the ideal food for these [premature] infants' being human milk—nature's food, certainly—but for the mature, healthy infant."[24] In other words, the authors of this study concluded that human milk was perhaps adequate for infants born healthy and full term but potentially dangerous for those in other conditions because of the slower growth patterns it produces. However, the line of reasoning that led to this scientific conclusion made sense only in the context of the much broader assumption underlying medical arguments at that time: the assumption that weight gain is the most important determinant of infant health. The medical emphasis on weight gain in mid-twentieth-century infant-feeding science was, in turn, related to other assumptions. Thus, for instance, one of the many assumptions that informed arguments about infant feeding in the mid–twentieth century was that protein levels are the most important aspect of infant-feeding substances. Rather than assuming human milk was the norm and that any artificial substance would probably fall short, the question was treated as open-ended, leaving physicians and scientists open to the possibility that an artificial substance might eventually achieve a level of protein superior to that in human milk. This was a situation that ultimately put those who would advocate the unique benefits of human milk and breastfeeding on the defensive.

This set of assumptions seems to have been widely shared among physicians who crafted arguments about infant feeding in the mid–twentieth century. The language used to distinguish breast- and bottle-feeding in a 1953 article offers further insight into how this conceptual framework operated: "It is a commonplace clinical observation that milk proteins supply a sufficient variety of amino acids to support growth in infancy. However, the optimum amount of protein for the growing infant is not known. This uncertainty is reflected in the wide range of protein content in the artificial milk formulas now offered for use."[25]

Attempting to contribute to the ongoing scientific conversation surrounding the nutritional adequacy of artificial substitutes, the article set out to address "the perennial question of maximal versus optimal nutrition."[26] The results of this study are not all that interesting from today's perspective, but the article is an important example because it illustrates the general conceptual framework in which mid-twentieth-century arguments about infant feeding were being made. Rather than assuming that human milk was the norm, or the standard that all artificial substances should be measured against, the topos breastfeeding as foundation left room for a suspicion that human milk might not measure up to artificial formulas derived from cow's milk. In fact, because cow's milk was known to contain higher protein levels than human milk and because artificial formulas appeared to produce faster infant weight gain, it seemed logical in this rhetorical situation to perceive human milk as inferior to the artificial formulas that scientists were continually working to improve.

The fact that this topos is evident in texts that offer clinical advice to health-care professionals who work with mothers, as well as in research articles, suggests how pervasive the notion of breastfeeding as foundation was in the mid-twentieth-century United States. It is important to acknowledge, however, that not everyone was fully on board with this understanding of the breast–bottle relationship. In fact, it was in 1956 that La Leche League was established to provide resources and support for mothers who wanted to breastfeed in spite of the many forces that were working to encourage bottle-feeding. For the most part, however, this organization and its followers existed in a marginal position outside of the medical community. They were available to assist those mothers who wanted to go out of their way to breastfeed successfully, but because the league founders were self-described laypeople rather than medical experts, they were not well positioned to exercise any influence over the medical community as a whole. It is notable that the pro-breastfeeding sentiments of the seven mothers who founded La Leche League were decidedly unscientific. As historian Julie DeJager Ward observes, the league founders supported "good mothering through breastfeeding," which is quite different from "simply saying that breastfeeding is a good choice backed up by sound reasons."[27] In short, science in the mid–twentieth century United States was on the side of the formula industry. Those who advocated breastfeeding—most notably La Leche League—were basing their claims on reasons not directly tied to scientific evidence. These nonscientific reasons produced arguments that were compelling to a passionately devoted segment of U.S. mothers who wanted to breastfeed and shared the league's narrow definition of good mothering as defined by breastfeeding. However, these arguments did not fundamentally alter the rhetorical framework in which arguments about infant feeding were made in the mid-twentieth-century United States, and that was a framework in which expert arguments were grounded in the topos of breastfeeding as foundation and science was decidedly on the side of those who advocated formula-feeding.

Late Twentieth Century:
The Topos of Breastfeeding as the Norm

Examining how the topos of breastfeeding as foundation framed the production of knowledge and arguments in mid-twentieth-century infant-feeding science and clinical practice provides a useful backdrop against which to understand the significance of the AAP's 1997 declaration that breastfeeding should be construed as "the reference or normative model against which all alternative feeding methods must be measured with regard to growth, health, development, and all other short- and long-term outcomes."[28] This 1997 statement, which has now been replaced by a 2005 revision that reinforces the same general stance, was important because it forcefully intervened in the ongoing discursive struggle to define what is normal. In so doing, the 1997 statement boldly and directly confronted the assumptions that governed infant-feeding research and clinical practice throughout much of the twentieth century. In fact, an important part of the exigency that demanded the 1997 policy statement was breastfeeding advocates' perception of the need for a document based on current scientific evidence about the health benefits of breastfeeding. The AAP's previous policy statement, which had been published in 1982,[29] cited very little evidence of this nature, even though such evidence did exist at that time. As a result, the traces of the topos of breastfeeding as a foundation on which infant-feeding decisions and practices are based are still evident in the 1982 statement. Specifically, the 1982 policy statement emphasized the "superiority of breastfeeding" but ultimately depicted infant feeding as a matter of individual choice.[30]

There was, however, a growing consensus in the mid 1990s that the AAP needed to update its stance and that the organization's new stance had to be clearly based on scientific evidence. Thus, for instance, minutes from the February 12, 1995, meeting of the AAP Work Group on Breastfeeding describe the policy statement that the work group envisioned at that time as "a more comprehensive, up-to-date statement with scientific documentation," and they assert that such a document "would be more appropriate and useful to the Academy and its membership" than the 1982 statement that the academy had just decided to retire.[31] As this statement indicates, there was an increasingly powerful commitment, at least among a certain contingency of AAP's membership, to the idea that science in the late twentieth century supported human milk's superiority over any artificial feeding substitute, but that medical policy and practice had not yet caught up with the latest scientific evidence.

This emphasis on scientific evidence is apparent in the final version of the AAP document published in 1997. The statement cites numerous research studies to document its claims about the health benefits of breastfeeding. The language of the statement uses this scientific evidence to ground its claim that breastfeeding should be treated as the normal infant-feeding method, rather than leaving open the possibility that formula might be superior in some respects. Specifically, the statement's second paragraph declares: "Human milk is uniquely superior for infant feeding and is species-specific; all substitute feeding options differ markedly from it. The breastfed infant is the reference or normative model against which all alternative feeding methods must be measured with regard to growth, health, development, and all other short- and long-term outcomes."[32]

The statement also spells out what should be expected as normal for the breastfeeding mother–baby pair. For instance, the statement provides a list of "Recommended Breastfeeding Practices," addressing matters such as feeding frequency for newborns, recommended weaning age, follow-up examinations for breastfeeding newborns discharged from the hospital, and introduction of solid foods. The list items instruct physicians as to how they might ensure that breastfeeding is treated as the norm in the clinics and hospitals where they practice medicine; these instructions are important because they suggest how health-care professionals might assist mothers to overcome breastfeeding problems rather than just implying that switching to formula is the best solution for most breastfeeding problems. In short, the 1997 AAP policy statement represents an important turning point in a decades-long history during which the topos of breastfeeding as foundation had spawned medical arguments that treated breastfeeding and medically supervised bottle-feeding as relative equals.

If the topography of the rhetorical landscape began to change in the 1990s, this is largely because breastfeeding advocates became able to make scientific arguments in favor of human milk's unique health benefits, and these arguments started to be convincing to increasingly broad audiences. (Although breastfeeding advocates had been engaged in rhetorical activity throughout the 1970s and 1980s, this activity had consisted primarily of economic arguments such as those that motivated the Nestlé Boycott and women's-rights arguments.)[33] The topos of breastfeeding as the norm first became publicly visible in the AAP's 1997 policy statement, but its formation was actually under way for many years before the policy statement appeared. For instance, in 1994 the AAP established a Work Group on Breastfeeding, and this was the group that eventually authored the 1997 statement. Also, in that same year, the Academy of Breastfeeding Medicine was established as "a worldwide organization of physicians dedicated to the promotion, protection and support of breastfeeding and human lactation."[34] The academy has been meeting at annual conferences since 1994 and has been publishing its own journal, *Breastfeeding Medicine,* since 2006. In other words, the 1997 policy statement did not necessarily announce new ideas; rather this statement stabilized and made official a set of ideas and knowledge that had been circulating in the pediatrics community for several years prior to 1997. In rhetorical terms, we might say these breastfeeding advocates' efforts helped to transform the emerging scientific ideas about human milk's unique health benefits into a topos that would mark a distinctive new shape in the rhetorical landscape of infant-feeding controversies.

Just as the topos of breastfeeding as foundation shaped the arguments that could be made about breast- and bottle-feeding in the mid–twentieth century, the topos of breastfeeding as the norm has begun to shape such arguments in recent decades. For example, in stark contrast to all of the earlier research that touted formula because it produced faster and greater weight gain in infants, today's medical discourse often emphasizes that it is normal for newborns to lose some weight in the first days after birth. Although newborns' weight patterns are still closely monitored by medical authorities, the weight-gain patterns of breastfed babies are now coming to be seen as normal, and, in fact, the AAP's 2005 policy statement cites nine studies to support its claim that breastfeeding might lead to a "reduction in incidence of . . . overweight and obesity."[35] Whereas medical researchers in the mid–twentieth century devoted most of their attention to determining how artificial substitutes might compensate for the perceived shortcomings in human milk, much of today's expert discourse on infant feeding seeks to perfect our understanding of the unique health benefits that human milk affords and to document these benefits with increasing levels of certainty.[36]

In the time that has elapsed since the AAP published its 1997 statement, then, the general trend in infant-feeding research has been to attempt to solidify the pro-breastfeeding stance by continuing to compile more evidence to document breastfeeding's unique health benefits and to deepen the divide between breast- and bottle-feeding. Although such evidence has continued to increase, there are also some experts who have called such evidence into question and have doubted the need for and appropriateness of distinguishing so sharply between breast- and bottle-feeding. In many ways, the strengthened pro-breastfeeding stance that was achieved in the 1997 statement and reinforced in the 2005 statement has changed the rhetorical topography by polarizing the breast–bottle controversy to a greater extent than it ever had been before.

Early Twenty-First Century:
The Topos of Formula as Risky

Whereas the topoi of breastfeeding as foundation and breastfeeding as the norm are quite clearly distinguishable from each other, the topos of formula as risky is best understood as an extension of the topos of breastfeeding as the norm. The formula as risky topos can be traced to the National Breastfeeding Awareness Campaign (NBAC), which began when the U.S. Department of Health and Human Services' Office of Women's Health was given funding to design a campaign that would work toward the breastfeeding goals outlined in the "HHS Blueprint for Action on Breastfeeding."[37] Specifically, the HHS Blueprint stated as a 2010 goal that 75 percent of U.S. mothers would breastfeed their babies in the early postpartum period and that 50 percent would still be breastfeeding at six months. Thus, in 2002 the Office of Women's Health partnered with the National Ad Council and McKinney & Silver LLC, a private advertising firm, to develop an advertising campaign whose goal would be "to increase awareness among women, their partners and families, employers and the community that breastfeeding is the ideal method of feeding and nurturing."[38] As a means of determining what would be the "most compelling triggers" for persuading U.S. mothers to breastfeed, a series of thirty-six focus groups was conducted in New Orleans, Chicago, and San Francisco. Because African American women have traditionally had lower breastfeeding rates than other U.S. demographic groups, the researchers made a special effort to target this audience by conducting half of the groups in each city with African American participants and the other half with non–African Americans. It was determined, through analysis of the focus-group results, that the most effective way to convince mothers to breastfeed would be to warn them about the dangers of infant formula.

Participants in these focus groups widely acknowledged that breastfeeding offers health benefits to the infant; from a rhetorical perspective, we might say the topos of breastfeeding as the norm that has dominated expert discourse since the 1990s also resonated with these focus-group participants. As noted in a presentation that reports the focus-group results, the "collective benefit of 'healthier baby' resonated more than any one isolated benefit," and "it appears that the 'System' has been effective in disseminating information about the positives."[39] However, those who analyzed the participants' responses surmised that most participants did not view these benefits as necessary; rather they tended to view human milk as something akin to a vitamin supplement. As the report notes, there was "a definite skew in language—breastfeeding is consistently spoken of in superlative terms like 'ideal or better,'" and "implicit in language is that breastfeeding compared to formula feeding is analogous to supplementing a 'standard diet' with more vitamins." Formula, by default, is credited with the status of being the "standard."[40] The researchers also determined that participants felt a great deal of fear and trepidation about breastfeeding because they expected to encounter many obstacles. In response to these findings, campaign designers determined that the only effective way to design messages that promote breastfeeding would be to use scare tactics—in other words, to emphasize formula as risky rather than just breastfeeding as healthy.

The Ad Council, along with McKinney & Silver LLC, acted on the focus-group findings by designing a comprehensive three-year media campaign that included a series of ads containing images such as an insulin syringe topped with a baby-bottle nipple and a baby bottle shaped as an asthma inhaler, suggesting that bottle-feeding is risky because it increases the risk of diabetes and asthma.[41] In November 2003, however, just before this massive campaign was scheduled to be broadcast, powerful formula-industry representatives who were present at the AAP's annual conference enlisted the AAP leadership to assist them in lobbying the government to stop them. On November 3, 2003, the same day that he was installed as AAP president, Dr. Carden Johnston was enlisted by formula-company representatives to sign a letter protesting the advertising campaign to Tommy Thompson, then secretary of the Department of Health and Human Services. What ensued was a heated yet short-lived debate that pitted formula-industry lobbyists and AAP leaders against breastfeeding advocates within the federal government and even within the AAP, where leaders and members of the AAP Section on Breastfeeding were outraged that their division had never been consulted regarding the letter sent to Tommy Thompson and endorsed by the AAP.[42]

Breastfeeding advocates who defended the campaign's content and tactics were accused of lacking objectivity, of basing the campaign on weak scientific evidence, and of using unethical scare tactics to persuade mothers to breastfeed. For instance, the letter that AAP president Dr. Johnston signed in protest to the campaign included the following language: "We note that the focus [of the campaign] will be on the risks incurred by not breastfeeding rather than to expound upon the benefits to be derived from breastfeeding. We have some concerns about this negative approach and how it will be received by the general public. . . . We must absolutely avoid making any claims that cannot be scientifically validated and thus undermine the credibility of the campaign."[43]

Advocates of the NBAC responded by accusing formula-industry representatives of having undue influence over the federal government and the scientific enterprise. They stood by the validity of the science on which the campaign was based and noted that similar tactics had been successfully used in a variety of other Ad Council campaigns. Most notably, Dr. Lawrence Gartner, who headed the AAP Section on Breastfeeding, included the following language in a letter he wrote in response to Dr. Johnston's letter: "We believe The Advertising Council's extensive experience in public service messages should be honored and followed. Many of their campaigns have had a major impact on improvement of health and social conditions for our citizens. Their PSA on Seat Belt Usage uses an approach similar to their plan for the Breastfeeding Campaign; they provide examples of what can happen when not wearing a seat belt."[44]

Eventually, in response to this pressure from the formula industry acting in conjunction with AAP leadership, the most dramatic advertisements were removed, and the campaign was substantially watered down. What was left in the campaign was a series of radio ads that targeted African American mothers in particular, some benign print advertisements that used images such as twin ice cream cones and pairs of dandelions positioned vaguely to resemble human breasts, and the shocking television commercials that depicted pregnant mothers riding mechanical bulls and participating in logrolling contests.[45] A *Los Angeles Times* article captures the way that many breastfeeding advocates felt about the outcome of this controversy: "It's a neat trick. The formula companies and their supporters have deftly reframed the debate. The science is invalid. So the debate isn't about science anymore, it's just about choice, and mothers shouldn't be made to feel guilty about their preferences."[46] Such a statement clearly points out how science serves as an ever-shifting frame in which the breast–bottle controversy unfolds.

Although the campaign's message was watered down, the message of formula as risky persisted in the NBAC television ads and might be said to constitute an emerging topos that could eventually result in a new scaffold for arguments about the relationship between breastfeeding and bottle-feeding. At the time of this writing, the notion of formula as risky has not been officially adopted in an AAP policy statement; the current AAP policy statement continues to emphasize the benefits of breastfeeding, not the dangers of formula-feeding. It is interesting, though, that the risks of formula-feeding are emphasized in a recent American Academy of Family Physicians position paper which says that "not breastfeeding is associated with increased risks of common conditions."[47] The topos of formula as risky is also apparent in promotional and informative materials of various nonmedical organizations. As just one example, the Florida Breastfeeding Coalition uses "The Cost of NOT Breastfeeding" as a heading on their website and includes information and links to other sites intended to help site visitors "KNOW the Difference between the BENEFITS of BREASTFEEDING and the RISK of FORMULA."[48]

Even as the topos of formula as risky continues to circulate, however, the efforts to refute breastfeeding advocates' scientific arguments continue to gain momentum. As Bernice L. Hausman observes, conflicting responses to the NBAC have centered on different responses to the scientific evidence on which the campaign is based.[49] Among those who have responded to the NBAC, feminist scholars have been some of the most vocal critics of the science that supports breastfeeding's superiority. For example, even before the NBAC controversy flared, Jules Law published an influential article that characterized scientific knowledge about the benefits of breastfeeding as subject to a great deal of uncertainty: "Quite simply, much (though certainly not all) of what has been written about the relative merits of breastfeeding and formula feeding is misleading at best and false at worst."[50] Law concludes, based on a review of some of the scientific literature that was available in the late 1990s, that "all too often, scientific research into the consequences and effects of infant-feeding choices concludes by acknowledging the inconclusiveness of its own results but then recommends breastfeeding on the grounds that its virtues are already well established in any case."[51] And, more recently, Joan B. Wolf has adopted an even stronger stance than Law, arguing that the current scientific research that experts use to demonstrate breastfeeding's superiority is fundamentally flawed. Wolf summarizes her main arguments as follows: "I argue that methodological and interpretive problems are pervasive at every step of the research process, from the design of their studies to the communication of their results; that as is often said, correlation does not equal causation; and that except in the case of gastrointestinal infections, the biological mechanisms by which breastfeeding promotes better health have not been demonstrated. In short, I contend that the unfounded certainty about breastfeeding's benefits in both scientific and popular culture is rooted in the discourse of breastfeeding research."[52]

Rebecca Kukla is another feminist scholar who has echoed Joan Wolf's criticisms. Kukla does not refute the scientific evidence as wholeheartedly as Wolf. In fact, Kukla notes some of the questions that remain unanswered in breastfeeding science, but, in contrast to Wolf, she believes that we do have adequate scientific evidence to support breastfeeding as an important public-health goal. As Kukla says, "we have enough unequivocal data about the benefits of breastfeeding to make it clear that achieving and maintaining high rates of initiating and continuing breastfeeding should be important public health goals."[53] Regardless of her faith in the quality and quantity of scientific evidence, Kukla still criticizes the NBAC because of the scare tactics that attempted to hold individual mothers responsible for failing to breastfeed without acknowledging the significant cultural obstacles that make breastfeeding so difficult for so many women.

A starkly different interpretation of current scientific evidence is evident in Jacqueline H. Wolf's feminist response to the NBAC controversy. In direct contrast to Jules Law, Joan Wolf, and Rebecca Kukla, Jacqueline H. Wolf outlines all of the reasons why we should accept the current scientific evidence in support of breastfeeding's health benefits and argues that feminists should be enraged that the formula industry's meddling in the breastfeeding-promotion campaign prevented U.S. women from receiving accurate information about the scientifically proven health benefits of breastfeeding.[54] Although Jacqueline Wolf acknowledges some good reasons why feminist scholars and activists might be reluctant to embrace breastfeeding as a political cause, she asserts that the controversy surrounding the NBAC "should have been condemned as evidence of what U.S. scientists charge is the Bush administration's suppression and distortion of science to further its political agenda."[55] Instead, she notes, feminist voices were largely absent from this controversy. Hausman makes a similar point, noting that feminist scholars who have criticized the NBAC after the fact have ended up taking the same side as formula-industry representatives. As Hausman says, "politics, in this case, did encourage the proverbial strange bedfellows."[56] It is hard to say what will be the eventual outcome of these feminist disagreements. In terms of a kairology of infant feeding, though, this ongoing controversy among feminist scholars reinforces the argument that the topoi of breastfeeding as the norm and formula as risky have enabled (and been enabled by) arguments in which science, at least for now, appears to be on the side of breastfeeding advocates. This rhetorical situation is, however, subject to change, especially if the efforts of those who are questioning the current scientific evidence continue to gain ground.

In examining this ongoing discussion, it is important to note that even when critics such as Law and Joan Wolf refute the scientific evidence that supports human milk's unique health benefits, they have not offered new evidence to take its place. This tendency is visible, for instance, in Joan Wolf's and Kukla's assertions that the currently available scientific evidence is not solid enough to warrant increasingly strident pro-breastfeeding messages such as those designed for the NBAC. Those who have argued from this perspective have not claimed to provide scientific evidence to show that formula-fed babies stand to gain some kind of health benefit that is not available to breastfed babies. A couple of recent scientific controversies, however, suggest that this feature of the current rhetorical topography is also subject to change. For instance, a few years ago there was some public attention to a resurgence of rickets among breastfed babies, purportedly occurring because the babies were not receiving adequate amounts of vitamin D in their mother's milk. Although only a small number of cases were reported, the issue received some media coverage, and breastfeeding advocates worried that this coverage would convey the message that human milk is deficient.[57] There has also been some recent attention to the risk of iron deficiency among breastfed infants, sparked by a 2010 *Pediatrics* article that reported on this potential health problem.[58] Whenever these controversies come up, we can see the fault lines that still exist within the AAP because spokespeople for the Section on Breastfeeding are quick to dispute any messages that come from other divisions of the organization if such messages might be used to judge breastfeeding as inferior or deficient. For instance, the AAP Section on Breastfeeding wrote an e-letter as a response to the report on iron deficiency, which had been authored by members of the AAP Committee on Nutrition. In their e-letter the authors who represent the Section on Breastfeeding say, in their opening line, "We have major concerns about universal iron supplementation at 4 months in breastfeeding infants."[59] As grounds for their concern, they call into question the research evidence that is cited in the report, noting that only one small study (involving only "77 breastfed term newborns") is cited and even questioning the relevance and strength of this small study's findings: "Follow-up studies found 'improved' psychomotor but not cognitive development at 13 months" in breastfed infants who received iron supplements. It is worth noting that the lead author of this e-letter, Richard J. Schanler, identifies himself as "FAAP Chairperson, AAP Section on Breastfeeding," and in the e-letter's last two paragraphs, the authors raise concerns about the truth of some of the claims that Baker and Greer's report on iron deficiency had made about endorsement by the AAP Section on Breastfeeding. As Schanler and his coauthors say: "Lastly, the authors acknowledge that this report was submitted for review to the Section on Breastfeeding of the American Academy of Pediatrics. It did not mention that we disagreed and provided our additional recommendations, 2 years ago. The manuscript infers that the Section, along with many other groups, endorsed this report. This is wrong and will mislead the medical community."[60]

Even though these issues regarding the potential for vitamin D and iron deficiency in breastfed infants have not achieved (at least not yet) the high public profile of the NBAC controversy, they are worthy of note because they suggest the extent to which the currently circulating topoi of breastfeeding as the norm and formula as risky are in flux because the scientific evidence used by those who build arguments from these topoi is continually subject to dispute. To the casual observer it might seem as if breastfeeding advocates are overreacting in the face of public messages such as these. But when we consider the larger rhetorical situation and history of anti-breastfeeding sentiments, their reactions make perfect sense. Along these lines, Hausman makes a convincing argument that when it comes to assessing risks, we live in a world in which most people are more likely to fear possible threats or contaminants in human milk than they are to fear health risks that might be incurred by formula-feeding.[61] Hausman's analysis is based on case studies of public fears about specific contaminants in human milk, including serious diseases such as HIV and West Nile virus, but she also discusses more general fears of contamination and impurity that seem to surface whenever we engage in public discussions about the maternal body and breastfeeding. Of course, the fears about vitamin D or iron deficiency in breastfed infants are more properly characterized as concerns about deficiency than about contamination or impurity per se. However, the divisions that surfaced within the AAP in response to these fears suggest a new trajectory for public discussions that would work against breastfeeding in a manner similar to the discourses on contamination and impurity that are the focus of Hausman's analysis. The public controversies that emerged because of these divisions within the AAP also suggest the potential for further changes in the rhetorical topography that situates our current understanding of the relationship between breast and bottle.

Where Are We Now?

The three different rhetorical commonplaces or topoi under review might be said to define "historical moments as rhetorical opportunities"[62] in U.S. infant-feeding policy and practice from the mid–twentieth century to the present. In the mid–twentieth century, U.S. pediatricians had come to understand breastfeeding as a foundation that designers of artificial substitutes should emulate. Toward the end of the twentieth century, the AAP adopted a quite different stance, declaring in their 1997 policy statement that breastfeeding is a normative model against which artificial substitutes should be measured. And finally, in the early twenty-first century, we are in the midst of a movement to establish formula as risky.

Echoing the comments of our focus-group participants who noted the importance of science in today's infant-feeding rhetoric, an important theme in this rhetorical history has been a decades-long shift in the ways that science is invoked by advocates of both breastfeeding and bottle-feeding. But adding some texture to these focus-group participants' remarks, the rhetorical history of infant-feeding discourse over the last several decades cannot be accurately understood as merely a story of scientific progress. Rather it is a story of shifting alignments and of the larger rhetorical framework in which infant-feeding science is conducted, produced, and disseminated. In the mid–twentieth century, science was undoubtedly on the side of the formula industry. Starting in the late twentieth century and continuing into the present, breastfeeding advocates have become increasingly able to use scientific evidence in ways that support a sharper distinction between human milk and formula. As this shift has occurred, it has been advantageous for breastfeeding advocates to frame the breast–bottle contest as one that can be decided by science—that is, scientific evidence that demonstrates health-providing qualities that are uniquely available in human milk. Indeed, as stated by Joan B. Wolf, our current rhetorical situation is characterized by "an overwhelming consensus that breastfeeding is the optimal form of nutrition for virtually all babies everywhere" and a "unanimity among health professionals" that breastfeeding is far superior to formula-feeding.[63] The emergence of the third topos, the notion of formula as risky, would seem to reinforce Joan Wolf's perceptions about the current rhetorical situation. On a broader cultural level, this topos would also seem to reflect a tendency that many scholars have noted to rely increasingly on the dictates of biomedical expertise in anticipation that our present behaviors can guarantee optimized future health for ourselves and for the children we care for.[64]

Because the notion of formula as risky is the newest of the three topoi, it is also the least clearly defined and its outcome is the most uncertain. As indicated by the controversy that flared around the NBAC, and the less visible recent controversies around risks of vitamin D and iron supplementation for breastfed babies, the apparent expert consensus in favor of human milk's unique health benefits is not as solid or unquestioned as it might seem. When we acknowledge expert controversies such as these, it becomes clear that the official medical consensus that "breast is best" does not tell the whole story of expert beliefs, scientific facts, and other rhetorical realities that shape infant feeding as a subject of medical expertise or as a lived, embodied experience for women in the United States today. In fact, even as the topos of breastfeeding as the norm has morphed into the stronger topos of formula as risky, the arguments of experts who advocate breastfeeding have been increasingly subject to attacks and refutations.

In short, although today's pro-breastfeeding rhetoric has considerable power, it is true also that the current rhetorical moment is unstable; conflicting beliefs and different types of information threaten to disrupt the seemingly smooth rhetorical topography defined by today's widely publicized medical consensus that "breast is best." Furthermore, although the three topoi under discussion have been presented as representing three distinct rhetorical moments, these topoi have not evolved from one to the next in a linear or progressive fashion, nor has each one replaced its predecessor. Rather, as new rhetorical commonplaces for understanding the breast–bottle relationship have come to exist, the old ones have lingered. The net effect is that all three ways of talking and thinking about the relationship between breast and bottle are still circulating today, and, as we shall see, each one is still accepted as true by some audiences in the contemporary United States, even though official medical and public-health texts continue to strengthen the language they use to articulate experts' support for breastfeeding. Carolyn R. Miller's observations about the intimate relationship between past and present in the concept of kairos might usefully illuminate this present situation. As Miller says: "Understanding the relationship between historical context and particular characteristics of discourse is essential to a specifically rhetorical interpretation of a scientific or any other text. . . . As the principle of timing or opportunity in rhetoric, kairos calls attention to the nature of discourse as event rather than object; it shows us how discourse is related to a historical moment; it alerts us to the constantly changing quality of appropriateness."[65] Thus, any effort to understand fully the kairos of the present moment in infant-feeding policies and practice must take these past commonplaces into account.

Acknowledging the nonlinear historical processes that have brought us where we are today and the conflicts that continue to exist behind the scenes of today's apparent pro-breastfeeding consensus are important steps toward providing a kairology of current U.S. infant-feeding policies and practices. Neither the recent history of U.S. infant-feeding discourse nor the current rhetorical topography is as smooth and uncomplicated as it might appear at first glance.

2

....

From "Wives' Tales and Folklore" to Scientific Fact

Rhetorics of Breastfeeding and Immunity
in the Mid-Twentieth Century

The idea that human milk affords the nursing infant a unique form of immune protection is not new. In fact, an immunology article published in 1988 cites an 1892 German study as the first to report that human milk affords some kind of immune protection.[1] A pediatrics article published in 1974 cites studies dated 1922, 1934, 1935, 1958, and 1961, all of which reported clinical results suggesting that breastfed babies fared better immunologically than their bottle-fed peers.[2] Despite this apparent cause-effect relationship, however, throughout much of the twentieth century the notion that breastfeeding might provide immune protection was perceived as mere speculation rather than scientific fact. As the introduction to a 1979 book entitled *Immunology of Breast Milk* explained, "both medical and veterinary scientists have long recognized the potential importance of immunity acquired after birth from the mother, although in clinical practice the arguments have often been accused of being wives' tales and folklore."[3]

In today's medical discourse, it appears that this old idea about human milk's immune protection has finally found its time—we might say it is the right kairotic moment for beliefs about human milk's immune protection to be accepted as scientific fact. For instance, the AAP's 1997 policy statement cites numerous studies to support the claim that breastfeeding protects against childhood diseases, including "diarrhea, lower respiratory infection, otitis media, bacteremia, bacterial meningitis, botulism, urinary tract infection, and necrotizing enterocolitis." The statement also cites studies that "show a possible protective effect" against several adult diseases, many of which are currently understood as related to the immune system, including "insulin-dependent diabetes mellitus, Crohn's disease, ulcerative colitis, lymphoma, allergic diseases, and other chronic digestive diseases."[4] The AAP's revised 2005 statement uses more definitive language and includes a longer list of infectious diseases than the 1997 statement. Specifically, the 2005 statement says: "Research in developed and developing countries of the world, including middle-class populations in developed countries, provides strong evidence that human milk feeding decreases the incidence and/or severity of a wide range of infectious diseases including bacterial meningitis, bacteremia, diarrhea, respiratory tract infection, necrotizing enterocolitis, otitis media, urinary tract infection, and late-onset sepsis in preterm infants."[5] Like the 1997 statement, the 2005 statement cites numerous scientific studies to support each of these claims.

Although both AAP policy statements cite a great deal of scientific evidence, the significant shift in medical beliefs that has occurred from the mid–twentieth century to the present has had little to do with scientific discoveries of new evidence about human milk's immune-protective properties. Rather, this shift in beliefs has occurred because a change in the metaphor that governs understandings of human immunity has produced a kairotic moment that is more amenable to scientific arguments in favor of human milk's immune protection. There has not been a particular scientific breakthrough or event that suddenly produced evidence so convincing that it definitively answered the long-standing question of whether or not human milk offers the infant immune protection. What has occurred is a more fundamental transformation in expert consensus about the essence of the object being studied, and that transformation has been possible because of a shift in the metaphor that shapes popular and scientific conceptions of human immunity.

To explore the rhetorical dimensions of this transformation, it is important to examine the scientific arguments about infant feeding and immunity that unfolded in key medical journals in the last half of the twentieth century. Our rhetorical analysis is based on close examination of fifty-nine articles from a wide range of pediatrics and immunology journals. To select these articles, I started by locating the key texts on infant feeding and immunity that the 1997 and 2005 AAP policy statements cite to justify their claims about the immune benefits of breastfeeding. From there, I worked backwards, attempting to locate any text cited as making a groundbreaking claim about infant feeding and immunity. Although research has led me to encounter a few publications that are much older, the majority of the articles were published from 1940 to 2005.

Closely examining the rhetorical transformation in beliefs about infant feeding and immunity that has occurred in this time span not only is an important first step toward understanding the kairos of the present moment in infant-feeding science but also has implications for feminist discussions of breastfeeding. Specifically, as we shall see, when human milk became recognized as part of the immune system, it was no longer seen as something unique to women's bodies. Instead it came to be seen as central to the human immune system, which has become a subject of intense scientific fascination in recent years. It is probably not purely coincidental that after this shift in perception of human milk's gendered dimension occurred, breastfeeding gained more respect in the medical community.

Shifting Metaphors of Human Immunity

As Donna Haraway observes, in the last quarter of the twentieth century the immune system became a "potent and polymorphous object of belief, knowledge, and practice" in scientific and popular understandings of bodies and selves.[6] The phenomenon that Haraway describes can be traced to 1954, when gamma globulin (an immune component of human blood) first became widely available to researchers. There was a corresponding explosion in scientific knowledge about the immune system. As Emily Martin explains, these findings continued to invigorate the field of immunology throughout the 1960s and 1970s, when a series of scientific breakthroughs further expanded scientific understanding of antibody function.[7] Because of the model that emerged through these discoveries, researchers began increasingly to idealize antibodies for their "flexible specificity."[8] Scientists who studied the immune system knew about the wide variety of antibodies before this time, and they knew that the body produced antibodies specific to different antigens, but the new model that emerged in the 1970s caused these traits to be further understood and emphasized. The belief entailed in this new model is that the body produces large numbers of antibodies to a wide variety of antigens, and when it encounters a particular antigen, it selects from this wide variety, and the antibodies specific to this antigen multiply.

Based on these fundamental changes in scientific understanding of antibodies, and drawing on recent developments in cybernetics and systems thinking, Martin characterizes late twentieth-century medicine and U.S. popular culture as moving from a "hierarchical machine" to a "complex-systems" metaphor of the immune system. In Martin's interpretation, the complex-systems metaphor entails a fundamentally different way of thinking about the body's ability to fight disease. Rather than viewing the immune system as located exclusively in the bloodstream and functioning to keep disease-causing agents out of the body, Martin says, the immune system in this new view is an integral part of a body capable of fighting disease at all of the body's surfaces—"a body that actively relates to the world, that actively selects from a cornucopia of continually produced new antibodies that keep the body healthy and enable it to meet every new challenge."[9] A complex system, as Martin describes it, consists of multiple feedback loops, so that instead of a centralized point of control, there are multiple points of control. Martin characterizes such systems as far less predictable than hierarchical-machine systems, in that "complex systems are extremely sensitive to fluctuation and change" in response to outside stimuli received by one or more parts of the system.[10]

The cultural shift that both Haraway and Martin discuss has been an important factor in the recent widespread acceptance of human milk's immune-protective qualities as scientific fact. To develop this argument, a chronological review will be useful, illustrating how the older "hierarchical-machine" metaphor shaped scientists' interpretations of data about infant feeding and immunity in mid twentieth-century research but how such interpretations gradually shifted throughout the last half of the twentieth century as the new "complex-systems" metaphor began to take hold. Although the complex-systems metaphor has played a central role in this process of fact construction, as one might imagine, metaphors do not emerge fully formed at a precise moment in scientific research; rather they constantly shift in response to new evidence at the same time as they actively shape how scientists interpret such evidence at any given moment.

Infant Feeding and Immunity
in the Mid-Twentieth Century

The mid–twentieth century in the United States has been characterized as an era of increasing faith in scientific solutions to problems, not only in the area of infant feeding but in other aspects of life as well.[11] Historians of medicine suggest that, corresponding to this demand for scientific solutions, many mid-twentieth-century physicians were eager to embrace bottle-feeding but also desired the kind of unequivocal scientific evidence that would finally settle the infant-feeding question that physicians had faced since the turn of the century when bottle-feeding began to rise in popularity and artificial formulas proliferated.[12]

Bo Vahlquist's 1958 review article "The Transfer of Antibodies from Mother to Offspring" provides a useful starting place for examining where research on infant feeding and immunity stood in relation to the mid-twentieth-century thirst for scientific answers. This article is significant because it seems to have offered a definitive answer to one of the many questions that researchers faced in this period: the question of whether the antibodies in human milk could be transferred from the mother to the nursing infant. In the article Vahlquist acknowledges that in many nonhuman species newborns receive antibodies through their mothers' colostrum and milk. However, he asserts that this is not the case in humans, and he firmly refutes other research-ers' claims to the contrary: "The essential features of antibody supply in many animal species differ from those of man, and disregarding this fact has led to many erroneous conclusions. A pertinent example is the false evaluation of the significance of colostrum and milk as vehicles for antibody supply to the human newborn."[13] Vahlquist's article proceeds by presenting an impres-sive amount of evidence demonstrating that antibodies from mother's milk can hardly ever be detected in more than trace quantities in the bloodstreams of nursing infants and, therefore, that human milk does not pass any signifi-cant amount of antibodies to the nursing infant. Vahlquist's claim that human milk could not afford immune protection was consistent with the hierarchical-machine metaphor of the immune system that dominated scientific thinking in this period. According to Martin, the hierarchical-machine metaphor entailed a view of antibodies as residing and enacting immune protection primarily in the blood system, and it did not account for the possibility of immune protec-tion operating in other bodily systems or fluids.[14]

Although Vahlquist's conclusions held a great deal of sway in the pediat-rics community for many years after they were published, his conclusions did not represent the only possible interpretation of the evidence. In fact, prior to Vahlquist's 1958 article, some researchers had already begun to look for a form of immune protection that human milk might offer through a means other than the bloodstream. For instance, a 1950 article reported that 80 per-cent of the human milk specimens in its study "contained varying amounts of neutralizing substance for the virus of poliomyelitis." Based on these find-ings, the authors of this article urged the medical community "to consider the role that breast feeding beyond the third month, or the drinking of 'antipolio-myelitic' cow's milk, might play in preventing or modifying the infection in human beings." Because the hierarchical-machine metaphor did not account for this type of antitoxic effect on bodily surfaces other than the bloodstream, the author of this article is careful to stipulate that the "antipoliomyelitic sub-stance in milk was not antibody."[15] Similarly, a 1955 article concluded that "milk (human, cow, goat) and human colostrum have a strong destructive factor against virulent and non-virulent mutants of leptospira."[16] Taking a slightly different approach but still reflecting the possibility of an unknown substance in human milk that enacts immune protection directly on multiple bodily surfaces, a 1953 article reported that the intestinal flora of breastfed infants consist mostly of Lactobacillus bifidus. This article then suggested that a particular "biochemical" substance in human milk promotes growth of this disease-fighting organism.[17]

Rhetorical scholars who have studied metaphor offer useful insights into the rhetorical situation that these mid-twentieth-century researchers faced in trying to present their dissenting views. Such theorists adopt the view that metaphor is intimately connected to knowledge construction. For instance, as Ken Baake suggests, when scientists encounter evidence that is not consistent with the dominant metaphor, they must "accommodate" the available language to make it correspond with the new evidence as closely as possible.[18] Along similar lines, Debra Journet concludes that the metaphors in the evolutionary biology texts she analyzes provide "a kind of disciplinary and interdisciplinary thinking tool that helps scientists 'grope' toward new understandings of the natural world."[19] And Evelyn Fox Keller makes the even stronger claim that metaphor and figurative use of language are central to the scientific endeavor:

> Scientific research is typically directed at the elucidation of entities and processes about which no clear understanding exists, and to proceed, scientists must find ways of talking about what they do not know—about that which they as yet have only glimpses, guesses, speculations. To make sense of their day-to-day efforts, they need to invent words, expressions, forms of speech that can indicate or point to phenomena for which they have no literal descriptors. . . . Making sense of what is not yet known is thus necessarily an ongoing and provisional activity, a groping in the dark; and for this, the imprecision and flexibility of figurative language is indispensable.[20]

As these theorists make clear, metaphor plays an especially important role in situations where scientific researchers encounter phenomena that cannot be explained by the currently available terminology.[21]

These theorists' observations about the role of metaphor in the production of new scientific knowledge are powerfully demonstrated in the language of mid-twentieth-century researchers who struggled to reconcile their findings with the hierarchical-machine metaphor. In an attempt to accommodate their findings to the dominant metaphor, such researchers described their findings in terms that now seem vague. The immune protection that they were witnessing seemed to depend on a loosely defined element that killed specific viruses and bacteria through direct contact, either in laboratory settings or on surfaces of the body such as the respiratory and digestive tracts.

These researchers' efforts to accommodate their findings to the dominant metaphor at the time apparently did not resonate well with their immediate audiences. Vahlquist's review article cites several such studies, and he says that their findings suggest a "local protective effect." However, Vahlquist quickly dismisses the possibility of such an alternative form of protection, stating simply that "the results of Sabin's experiments to show such a local effect in the digestive tract have not been unequivocal."[22] Vahlquist then moves on to offer readers additional evidence against the idea that human milk affords immune protection.

Resisting Vahlquist
....

Vahlquist's 1958 review article was significant not because it presented new evidence but because it presented large amounts of data accumulated over several decades in an argument that seemed, at least temporarily, to satisfy the medical community's desire for definitive answers to the infant-feeding and immunity question. However, in establishing such a strong and well-accepted argument, Vahlquist also provided the rhetorical target at which anyone who wanted to argue for breastfeeding's immune benefits would aim for years to come. In rhetorical terms, Vahlquist's article played an important role in establishing a stasis that defined infant-feeding research throughout the 1960s and 1970s and was eventually unsettled in the 1980s. Stasis is, defined simply, "the place where rhetoric begins, an explicit or implicit disagreement or conflict."[23] In science, stasis can be understood as the unresolved issues or tensions that scientists agree are at the heart of their quest for knowledge at any given moment, as a "'gap' in certifiable knowledge" or a "point . . . that must be settled somehow before any further progress can be made in discussing the overall problem."[24]

Thus, to say that Vahlquist's 1958 text defined a stasis is to say that it articulated one of the burning questions that his contemporaries were asking and also that it established the "point of stoppage" that subsequent researchers would encounter when they made arguments in response to this question. This point is further clarified by John T. Gage's observation that the "situations of conflict of knowledge" that constitute points of stasis "are the mutual invention of the writer and the audience."[25] In other words, a stasis does not exist entirely independent of the moves of a rhetor such as Vahlquist; rather, it is, in part, shaped by such moves.

Because of the stasis that Vahlquist's 1958 article helped to solidify, his article made it much more difficult for later researchers to convince the pediatrics community that the antibodies in human milk were providing significant immune protection. However, researchers did not stop looking for evidence of immune protection altogether; they simply had to intensify the effort to find a different kind of immune protection. Using various approaches, authors who published new findings in the 1960s and 1970s began to pay more attention to the speculation that Vahlquist's article had mentioned but swiftly dismissed: the possibility that milk antibodies exercise local rather than systemic immune protection by resisting antigens directly on the surfaces of the digestive tract.

The situation that these researchers faced was made easier by some findings that immunologist Lars A. Hanson reported in 1961 and 1962. In a 1961 article, Hanson identified a type of antibody in human milk that he suggested might function differently from the serum antibodies that medical researchers were accustomed to studying.[26] In some ways, Hanson's article does not seem much different from the 1950s articles in which authors hypothesized the existence of a local immune protection operating on bodily surfaces other than the bloodstream. Like the authors of these earlier articles, Hanson used currently available terminology to accommodate his findings to the dominant metaphor at the time, which dictated that gamma globulin was the primary vehicle for immune protection. He called the antibodies he identified "gamma-globulins of milk."

However, in Hanson's study we see the significance of interdisciplinary approaches to research problems. As an immunologist, he went further than previous pediatrics researchers had gone in speculating about the differences between milk and serum antibodies and the mechanisms underlying such differences. Although his language was still imprecise and speculative, Hanson suggested that milk antibodies might be "serum antibodies to some extent modified in the mammary gland" and that the "difference between the antibodies in serum and milk could be important in relation to the absorption of immune globulins from the gut of the breast-fed child."[27] Hanson's language anticipated the unpredictable, multiple, and nonlinear way of thinking about the immune system that would accompany the new complex-systems metaphor immunologists came to embrace more fully in the 1970s.

Perhaps because Hanson was an immunologist rather than a pediatrician, his are some of the few post-1958 publications considered in this chapter that did not cite Vahlquist. This point is significant not only because it altered the rhetorical situation that surrounded Hanson's arguments, but also because it changed the essence of the object that he and other researchers were studying. Offering a glimpse of a situation that bears some resemblance to this situation, Annemarie Mol's ethnographic study of atherosclerosis as it was "enacted" in different units of specialization within a single hospital suggests that "different enactments of a disease entail different ontologies." In other words, according to Mol, the pathologist examining blood vessels in an amputated leg is actually dealing with a different ontological entity than the clinician who seeks to treat the pain that the patient is experiencing, and the surgeon who might operate on or amputate the affected leg is dealing with yet another entity. Each of these specialists might perceive themselves as treating or diagnosing the same disease. However, as Mol says, "they each do the body differently. . . . In each variant of atherosclerosis the dis of this dis-ease is slightly different."[28] From this perspective, we might surmise that immunologists studying human milk in the 1960s were studying an entity different from that examined by pediatrics researchers who had accepted Vahlquist's assertion that human milk did not afford immune protection. In this case, the new disciplinary perspective of immunology researchers drastically altered how human milk would be understood in subsequent research.

In a 1962 follow-up to his 1961 article, Hanson and collaborator Bengt G. Johansson added further credence to Hanson's initial speculations. They did so by reporting the results of their successful attempt to isolate human milk antibodies "in order to examine more closely the relationship between the immune globulins of milk and of blood serum."[29] In particular, the researchers reported that they had isolated a milk antibody that they called milk β_{2A}—globulin—the existence of which was first postulated in Hanson's 1961 article. Although this milk antibody was still not understood as precisely as it would be later, the 1962 article was important because it used an imaging technique called immune electrophoresis to confirm what had merely been suspected in the 1961 article: that antibodies unique to human milk do exist and that they behave somewhat differently from serum antibodies.

As Bruno Latour and Steve Woolgar observe, the type of isolation and identification that can be accomplished by images such as those in Hanson and Johansson's 1962 article are important steps in the production of scientific truth. Such images are important because once a hypothesized substance has been identified and isolated, researchers can stop devoting energy to disputing its existence and nature, and they can instead use it as a "tool." Once this happens, the substance "provides one less concern, or one less source of noise, for the researcher."[30] In other words, isolation and identification of a substance can contribute to the construction of scientific facts by causing researchers' speculations to converge around a belief or set of beliefs that are increasingly certain, rather than to continue moving in various directions.

Latour and Woolgar's insights about the rhetorical importance of scientific images usefully illuminate the trajectory that research on breastfeeding and immunity followed throughout the 1960s and 1970s. After the electrophoretic images that Hanson and Johansson published in 1962, researchers finally had laboratory evidence for an immune component in human milk, rather than just clinical evidence, and consequently they were able to develop more precise scientific arguments with regard to this component. In the work that such researchers accomplished with the new "tool" available to them, we see how an emerging metaphor can generate knowledge by causing scientists to see old evidence in productive new ways. Specifically, after these breakthroughs in immunology, human milk gradually became associated with the complex-systems metaphor of the immune system that, in Martin's interpretation of history, was beginning to emerge in the 1960s and became more fully formed in the 1970s.[31]

As this association continued to develop, researchers gained access to a new vocabulary, and along with this vocabulary came a new framework for interpretations of evidence related to the question of human milk's immune protection. Even though the researchers who challenged Vahlquist's 1958 conclusions continued to cite his article, they could grant his claims a much narrower scope than Vahlquist himself had done. Moreover, with the precise scientific terminology that became available as the new complex-systems metaphor emerged and began to gain momentum, these researchers were eventually able to unsettle the stasis that Vahlquist's article had established. Thus, the power of Vahlquist's broad-sweeping claim against human milk's immune-protective qualities diminished throughout the next couple of decades as pediatrics researchers came to restate it in increasingly narrow terms and to place greater emphasis on the local, rather than systemic, immune protection offered by human milk.

We begin to see this effect in a 1967 article titled "Bacterial and Viral Coproantibodies in Breast-Fed Infants."[32] Like many other pediatrics texts in this period, the article cited Vahlquist's 1958 review article in its opening paragraph to support the following synopsis of previous research: "The existence of bacterial and viral antibodies in human milk has been known for some time. However, since most investigators have found that little parenteral absorption occurs in the human being, these antibodies generally have been considered unimportant in the immune system of the newborn infant."[33] The authors of this article then proceed to resist the previously accepted "fact" about the role of antibodies in human milk, citing Hanson and Johansson's 1962 publication to support their claim that human milk might "offer some degree of immunity to intestinal infections during early infancy."[34] In search of evidence for this kind of protection, the authors conducted a study that looked for coproantibodies, which means antibodies in the stools of newborn breast-fed infants rather than in the blood. They found evidence of such antibodies, and they confirmed that such antibodies came from mother's milk because "titers of antibody in infant feces correlated well with those in the mother's milk."[35] Furthermore, the researchers ruled out "serum as a direct source of fecal antibody" by noting little correlation between antibody levels in mother/infant serum and those in infant stool. As further evidence for their claim, they noted that such antibody activity was not found in the stools of bottle-fed infants.

As we see in this article's "Comment" section, these authors' more definitive arguments became possible because, as human milk came to be associated with the newly emerging idea of an alternative, supplementary immune system, it also came to be affiliated with a metaphor that could compete with the hierarchical-machine metaphor that underlay Vahlquist's 1958 claims. Reflecting the move toward what Martin calls the "complex-systems" approach to thinking about the immune system, in its "Comment" section the article on coproantibodies echoed Hanson's earlier speculations about the existence of an additional, previously undiscovered immune system that operates in a self-regulating manner in response to specific stimuli that the intestinal cells encounter: "Antibody appears earlier in intestinal mucus than in serum, suggesting that the intestine has an immune system of its own with cells which may produce antibody following local antigenic stimulation."[36]

The momentum toward such an alternative, supplementary immune system continued to build in research on human milk conducted throughout the 1970s. For instance, a 1971 article that cited both Vahlquist and Hanson, as well as the above-mentioned article on coproantibodies, reported on a study of ninety-nine infants, including thirty-three who were infected with neonatal meningitis or urinary tract infections and sixty-six uninfected controls. The researchers concluded that those infants in the study who had consumed the most human milk were the least likely to be infected. The authors connected this finding to the emerging idea of human milk as a source of local protection: "These antibodies [in human milk] are probably not absorbed, but their presence in colostrum and their ability to pass through the gut with well-retained antibody activity would accord with a role in local defence against E. coli."[37] Next these authors repeated the speculation that multiple systems might work together to fight infection in the newborn. The language of their speculation echoes the move toward associating breastfeeding with the complex-systems metaphor of the immune system: "Thus there might be a defence against gramnegative septicaemia at several levels—one local . . . the other humoral. . . . Obviously other defence systems are present."[38]

It is interesting that this 1971 article cited Vahlquist's 1958 article as the single source for its claim that "these antibodies [in human milk] play little if any, role in man's humoral defence," but it then went on to position its hypothesis relative to Vahlquist's stance: "But since some of them are passed along the intestinal tract with activity intact they may have local effects."[39] The authors later cited Vahlquist again as a source for the following statement: "These antibodies are probably not absorbed," and they again contrasted their own findings to Vahlquist's established fact: "but their presence in colostrum and their ability to pass through the gut with well-retained antibody activity would accord with a role in local defence against E. coli."[40]

Articles throughout the 1970s continued to produce further evidence for the assertion that human milk affords local protection and, more important, that this local protection is an integral part of an immune system consisting of multiple components that work together to fight infection on multiple fronts. An article that included Hanson as one of its coauthors provides a good indication of the status of beliefs about infant feeding and immunity at the beginning of the 1970s. Published in 1972, the article reflected back on the significance of

Hanson and Johansson's 1962 findings and explicitly connected these findings to the new understanding of breastfeeding and immunity that the pediatrics community would later adopt. The article began by noting that newborns in the 1970s were being exposed to more disinfectants and antibiotics and less breastfeeding than ever before. The authors then observed: "The fact that this trend has continued side by side with a situation where infections have played a diminishing role in neonatal morbidity and mortality has created the impression that such changes have been beneficial, or at least not harmful, to the infant."[41] The article then provided evidence of the long-standing influence of Vahlquist's article in perpetuating doubt about human milk's immune benefits. The manner in which the authors refer to Vahlquist's article confirms that the 1962 isolation and identification of human milk antibodies had played a central role in enabling researchers to overcome Vahlquist's truth claims: "The possible role of the low consumption of breast milk has attracted little attention, and historically the fact that the antibodies of milk are not absorbed from the gut in the human (Vahlquist, 1958) is perhaps partly responsible for this. With the appreciation of secretory IgA as the main immunoglobulin in breast milk, and also as an important immune factor for epithelial surfaces, a new situation has developed. This, as well as the recognition of several other antibacterial factors in breast milk, has reopened discussion of the value of breast milk."[42] However, despite this apparent increase in certainty, the article's conclusion was still cautious in making claims about human milk's immune protection, and it ended with a call for more research.[43]

Thus, a full decade after Hanson and Johansson's 1962 identification and isolation of milk antibodies, researchers still perceived a need for more scientific research and rhetorical work to convince scientific and medical audiences that the 1962 evidence was relevant to the infant feeding and immunity question. Although researchers who believed in human milk's immune-protective qualities were using the important new evidence from immunology to strengthen their argument that human milk provided local protection, they could not refute Vahlquist's 1958 truth claims all at once because the complex-systems metaphor of the immune system had not yet fully entered into these researchers' interpretive framework.

Shortly after Hanson and Winberg's 1972 article, however, a handful of publications started to assume a more definitive stance. This more definitive stance was clearly connected to the fact that the complex-systems metaphor for the immune system was gaining ground as the field of immunology continued to explode. For instance, a commentary by John W. Gerrard says, with regard to the challenge that recent immunological research was posing to Vahlquist's 1958 article, that Vahlquist's "review of the passage of immunoglobulins from mother to fetus, written before the recent explosion of information on the structure and function of immunoglobulins, stated that the fetus derived all of his immunologic protection transplacentally and that, though some immuno-globulin was present in colostrum, this was of no clinical consequence."[44]

Gerrard then proceeded to counter Vahlquist's well-established truth claim and to urge the pediatrics community to join him in rethinking long-standing medical beliefs about infant feeding and immunity: "Most of us in the prac-tice of pediatrics, as in so many other areas, have taken a permissive attitude toward breast-feeding. This attitude is understandable, since we presumed that the function of breast milk was little more than the provision of nourishment. We now know that breast milk also provides effective protection, more effec-tive than antibiotics, against certain common enteric pathogens, and that it can also be expected to provide relative freedom in infancy from allergic disease, a growing problem of modern feeding habits."[45] Gerrard's remarks indicate that the stasis or "point of stoppage" that Vahlquist's 1958 review article had played such an important role in establishing was, by the mid-1970s, well on its way to being unsettled. This unsettling coincided with a period during which the new knowledge resulting from the rapid expansion of immunology continued to infiltrate pediatrics researchers' understanding of infant feeding and immunity.

Three years after Gerrard's commentary was published, an immunology article cited Hanson and Winberg's 1972 article to support the following claim: "Human colostrum and milk has now been shown to possess a wide variety of host-resistance factors." This 1977 article seems to dismiss Vahlquist's findings altogether. It is interesting that the authors did not cite him and that their arti-cle contains the following sentence: "Although in many mammalian species, the absorption of immunoglobulin in the intestine is well established and often constitutes the sole source of passive immunity in the neonatal period [the authors cite several studies here], the data on intestinal absorption of immu-noglobulin in man are too fragmentary and conflicting."[46] The article then concluded "that breast feeding during the 1st week after the onset of lactation may be crucial in providing the infant with immunologically active ingredients in a concentrated form at a time when the mechanisms of mucosal defense are less than optimal."[47]

Suggesting that the stasis established by Vahlquist's 1958 article had been altered even further by the 1980s, a 1986 pediatrics article began by citing Vahlquist as the source of the following claims, which the authors felt confi-dent in portraying as outdated: "The presence of immunoglobulins in breast milk was initially thought to have no significance for infants. It was believed that all immunologic protection in the human neonate was acquired transpla-centally."[48] The article then went on to cite several recent studies that refuted Vahlquist by demonstrating the significance of the unique kind of antibody human milk contains. Based on this evidence, the authors concluded that "it is now generally accepted that human milk affords the infant primarily enteric protection, whereas systemic immunity is enhanced by transplacental passage of immunoglobulins."[49] The article also stated what was emerging as the new view of human milk: "Because artificial replication of these species-specific immunity factors is not possible currently, breast milk remains unique when compared with prepared formulas."[50] This same article also emphasized the centrality of the new understanding of immunity to the emergence of the new view of breastfeeding: "The ability of breast milk to confer passive immunity has withstood the test of time well and remains the leading impetus to encourage breast milk feedings."[51]

Metaphor and Interdisciplinary Harmonics

The only piece of evidence that might be considered new in the story of scientific progress reviewed so far is Hanson and Johansson's 1962 electrophoretic images of the immune-protective elements in human milk. However, this piece of evidence did not single-handedly or instantaneously change researchers' beliefs; it took more than a decade after Hanson and Johansson's images for researchers to start talking about human milk's immune benefits as scientific fact. In other words, neither the new metaphor nor the new evidence emerged fully formed at a precise moment. Rather, the relationship between the two has always been in flux—the metaphor shifting ever so slightly as scientists used language to accommodate new evidence and also shaping how scientists interpret such evidence at any given moment. In fact, the term *metaphor* derives from the Greek words *epiphora* and *phora*, which both imply movement, and "such movement suggests that truth can never be fixed in language, but must be constantly renegotiated (constructed) as new metaphors appear."[52] Lending support to this notion of a dynamic relationship between new evidence and the metaphors that govern its interpretation, new scientific evidence about human milk's immune-protective qualities has been so closely intertwined with changing metaphors of the immune system that it is impossible to pinpoint an exact moment when the truth changed or a place where science ends and rhetoric begins in this narrative of scientific progress.

To understand the significance of Hanson and Johansson's 1962 evidence in unsettling the stasis that Vahlquist's 1958 article established, we have to look beyond the evidence itself and consider the larger context that surrounded it. This enlarged perspective reveals that the images were an important piece of evidence not only within the narrow confines of infant-feeding science but also because they coincided with a larger explosion of scientific knowledge about the immune system in general. With this explosion of knowledge, the human immune system became an increasingly important object of scientific study throughout the time frame under consideration. In fact, the number of researchers in immunology was 10,000 in 1970, compared to only 3,300 in 1950 and 110 in 1930.[53] Although it would be difficult to obtain an exact count of how many of the 10,000 immunology researchers in 1970 were specifically focusing their efforts on human milk, the following paragraph from the introduction to a 1979 book entitled *Immunology of Breast Milk* suggests that human milk occupied a prominent position in the spotlight that was cast by the explosion of knowledge about the immune system that began in the 1950s and gained momentum throughout the 1960s and 1970s: "Although the predominance of IgA in human colostrum and milk had been described, the importance of this observation was not fully appreciated until the discovery that IgA was a predominant immunoglobulin class in a variety of mucosal secretions in addition to breast milk. This set the stage for the explosion of knowledge concerning mucosal immunity that has accumulated over the past 15 years."[54] This language suggests that Hanson and Johansson's evidence was important because it caused human milk to become associated with the newly emerging metaphor of the immune system that was causing so much excitement for immunology researchers.

Hanson et al. said in a 1988 article that looked retrospectively at the recent history of developments in understanding human milk's immune protection that "only when the special characteristics of sIgA antibodies in milk and other external body fluids were discovered was it realized that these antibodies were to function on mucosal membranes, not in tissues." The authors summarized these "special characteristics" as follows: "The main function of SigA antibodies is to bind antigens. The most important function in host defense is presumably to bind bacteria preventing them from attaching to mucosal membranes, an important first step in the initiation of most infections. The antibodies in milk against bacterial adhesins, such as pili or fimbria, may mediate such anti-adherence activity."[55] Hanson et al.'s description of how the immune-protective elements in human milk function clearly reflects the phenomenon to which Martin refers when she says that biomedical discourse has moved toward a model of the human immune system as "flexibly specific."

The language that Hanson and his coauthors used also reflects the shift to what Martin called a "complex-systems" metaphor of the human body, and the authors embraced the new metaphor with more certainty than the authors of any of the previous texts we have examined. For instance, in summarizing recent advances in understanding the immune functions of human milk, these authors referred to research that "demonstrated the presence of an entero-mammaric pathway of lymphoid cells homing to the mammary glands after antigenic exposure in the Peyer's patches in the intestine."[56] In other words, through this enteromammaric pathway, antigens to which the infant's intestine is exposed cause the mother's mammary glands to produce antibodies specifically designed to fight against them. Additionally, the authors pointed to a study that suggested the existence of a "bronchomammaric pathway" that functions in a similar way to produce and deliver to the infant antibodies against antigens that affect the respiratory system.

Thus we can conclude that the rise of the complex-systems metaphor allowed researchers in the 1970s gradually to reject Vahlquist's 1958 version of the truth. One reason the shift happened is that human milk suddenly became affiliated with a different sphere of research—immunology rather than pediatrics—and this new sphere of research was being invigorated in productive new directions by the rise of a new metaphor. In rhetorical terms, the movement facilitated by the metaphor unsettled the stasis (which means "stoppage point" or lack of movement) that had circumscribed infant-feeding debates for several decades prior to this time. Specifically, when human milk became affiliated with the emerging metaphor of the complex system, pediatrics researchers were able to make more convincing arguments about it. This affiliation forced medicine to adopt a more expansive view of human milk; rather than merely a feeding substance whose nutritional qualities could presumably be reproduced in an artificial substance, it came to be more highly respected as an object of scientific research.

From a feminist perspective, it is significant that this new understanding entailed a shift from a view in which human milk was seen primarily as a component of women's reproductive systems (and not a very important component insofar as it was increasingly seen as one that could be replaced by an artificial substitute) to a view of it as a central component of the human immune system. It is interesting to note that in research articles published prior to this shift in perspective, human milk and human lactation were routinely compared to their animal equivalents. For instance, Vahlquist's 1958 conclusions were based on a synthesis of dozens of studies, many of which explicitly compared human colostrum and milk to the colostrum and milk from various animal species, including cows, lambs, pigs, and rodents. In all of the studies that Vahlquist cited, human colostrum and milk compared unfavorably to the animal substances. As just one example, Vahlquist made the following comparison between human and cow colostrum: "In the woman the amount of colostrum is small, on the average not over 100 Gm. in the first 3 days postpartum (about 30 Gm. per kilogram of the offspring's body weight). In comparison, the cow produces 30 Kg. during the 3 days, or about 1,000 Gm. per kilogram body weight of offspring. Furthermore, the antibody concentration in bovine colostrum is often many times that in human colostrum."[57]

In addition to the numerous studies on immunity that Vahlquist cited, there exist enough other articles making explicit comparisons between human lactation and animal lactation to suggest that this was a persistent tendency in mid-twentieth-century medical research. One of these began by citing previous research on the let-down function in cows: "As a result of considerable investigation by Petersen and others [3 studies cited here] in cows, the mechanism can be postulated as follows."[58] The authors use this reference to previous research on the let-down reflex in cows as a prelude to stating their own research question, which addresses the let-down reflex in lactating women: "The let-down reflex has long been recognized as an important factor in the success of milking cows. The purpose of this paper is to investigate whether it is an important factor in the success of lactation in women."[59] Another article began with the observation that "it has been known for some time that in cows the number of milkings in 24 hours influences milk production," and then moved on to make a similar observation about human lactation: "In human beings, Macy et al., . . . showed that milk production rose when the breast was emptied five or six times daily."[60]

The fact that all of these comparisons between human and animal milk seemed to diminish when human milk started to be seen as a component of the immune system, rather than simply a part of women's reproductive function, should not go unnoticed by feminist scholars who are interested in the current discourses of infant feeding. Although there is not anything blatantly sexist or misogynistic in such historical examples of seemingly neutral scientific prose, it is concerning from our contemporary perspective to see human milk (a substance that is only produced by the female body and is affiliated with women's reproductive systems) repeatedly compared—usually in an unfavorable light—to similar substances and processes in a variety of animals. As Londa S. Schiebinger notes, Western science has a long history of equating women's reproductive functions, especially lactation, with animals, whereas other characteristics affiliated with maleness or perceived as gender neutral (such as intelligence and rationality) are used to distinguish humans from animals.[61]

Implications for a Kairology of Infant Feeding

Beginning with Martin's observation that the complex-systems metaphor for the immune system emerged gradually in immunology research throughout the last half of the twentieth century,[62] we have looked at how this metaphor emerged and developed alongside new scientific facts about breastfeeding and immunity. The analysis tells a story of scientific "progress" that is not about rhetoric, science, or medicine but about the complex intersections among these domains. In this story, the discovery of new evidence is intertwined with the rhetoric surrounding it in such a way that neither makes sense apart from the other. Specifically, although it had long appeared that breastfeeding enhanced immunity, this cause-effect relationship was not treated as scientific fact until the dominant metaphor of immune protection could account for an immune system operating in parts of the body other than the bloodstream. At the same time, though, this larger shift in the metaphor that governs understandings of the immune system was made possible only through years of scientific research on the immune system.

As the medical historian Paul Starr observes, the history of infant feeding in the United States is an area in which it could be argued that medical progress has done more harm than good.[63] From Starr's perspective, the recent explosion of medical knowledge about breastfeeding has paradoxically produced scientific "progress" only by pushing medical attitudes back to what they were more than a century ago, before commercially produced formulas were widely available. The detailed picture we have drawn of the scientific events that Starr criticizes is important for several reasons.

First, from the perspective of medical-practice guidelines, the shift in beliefs that has resulted from increased understanding of human milk's immune qualities has given valuable support to the small minority of people in the medical community who had long believed in the advantages of breastfeeding over bottle-feeding. The experts who wrote about and researched infant feeding in the mid–twentieth century had always been able to justify ambivalence toward breastfeeding by claiming that there was a lack of certain knowledge: there were no facts to prove human milk's superiority, so medical discourse would not take a definitive stance in support of breastfeeding and instead perpetuated the idea that formula is, or eventually could be, an equivalent substitute. As we shall see, the increased medical understanding of how antibodies in human milk operate has helped breastfeeding advocates argue convincingly that human milk cannot be replaced by any artificial substitute. This new understanding poses a serious challenge to the topos of breastfeeding as foundation because it refutes the long-standing assumption that the food women's bodies could provide to their infants was less than perfect, and therefore could be imitated and even improved upon through scientific research. The new medical perception of breastfeeding also resonates with popular images of health and wellness, which, Martin observes, have come to be understood as dependent on a well-functioning immune system: "The underlying common regard for the immune system in our culture allows it to become a kind of currency in which health—degrees of it—can be measured and compared among different people and populations."[64] In fact, Martin mentioned in passing that breastfeeding is one of several examples of "phenomena [that] have been given new interpretations and understandings" as the immune system has become more deeply entrenched in our collective understandings of the body and diseases that threaten it.[65]

Second, in addition to contributing to a historical understanding of scientific beliefs about human milk and immunity, our historical analysis also suggests some important gendered dimensions of recent breastfeeding discourse that feminist scholars have not yet identified.[66] Contrary to what many feminist scholars suggest, we have seen that the new medical support of breastfeeding has actually come about through rhetorical moves that disarticulate breastfeeding from women's reproductive functions and articulate it more closely with the presumably gender-neutral human immune system. This means it is inaccurate to argue, as many feminist scholars have, that the current medical enthusiasm for breastfeeding is motivated by a desire to return to traditional ideologies of biological mothering.[67] The observation that human milk has begun to receive more respect within medical circles since its immune-protective functions have come to be more fully understood is important, then, because it shows how a rhetorical analysis can complicate current feminist critiques of breastfeeding discourse and can help us achieve a more nuanced understanding of the ways in which such discourse relates to contemporary understandings of gender differences.

As feminist scholars Emily Martin and Lisa Adkins have both observed, the rise of complex-systems metaphors and the idealization of traits such as flexibility that has accompanied this larger shift in how we think about the human body, health, and sickness have important implications for late twentieth- and twenty-first-century understandings of gender.[68] Although, as Martin observes, many of the changes seem favorable to women's bodies, we also have to beware, as Adkins argues, that such changes can follow a trajectory that is ultimately unpredictable: gender binaries might be reversed, but this type of reversal seldom has a predictable outcome. Thus, the recent shift in how the medical community perceives human milk and lactation still might raise concerns from a feminist perspective, but these are different concerns, and probably more complex, from those emphasized by current feminist critics. Finally, our rhetorical analysis provides a useful reminder that the facts communicated to lay audiences on subjects such as infant feeding are usually more subject to scientific debate than the decisive tone of medical-advice literature might suggest. The certainty with which facts about human milk's immune-system benefits are presented today might easily obscure the fact that human milk's immune-protective qualities have been one of the most hotly contested subjects in experts' discussions about infant feeding during the last several decades. And, in fact, even as they have begun to gain ground in the pediatrics community, beliefs in human milk's immune-protective qualities have not stood unchallenged, just as Vahlquist's 1958 conclusions were not unchallenged in their own time. For instance, a 1984 supplement to the journal *Pediatrics* reported a great deal of evidence showing that, although the immune-protective benefits of breastfeeding are essential in some parts of the world, they are not as essential in developed countries where higher hygiene standards, health-care quality, and availability of antibiotics can compensate for such benefits.[69] Thus, in light of our insights into the complex relationships among science, medicine, and rhetoric, perhaps the recent medical endorsement of human milk's immune-protective qualities is most accurately understood as indication that a certain set of ideas has won out for the moment, not that the long-lasting medical debate over infant feeding has come to an end.

3

....

Articulating Knowledge and Practice

The Rhetoric of Infant-Feeding Policy

We now take a more in-depth look at the three AAP policy statements that have communicated the organization's official stance on breastfeeding during the last three decades. The first statement, titled "The Promotion of Breastfeeding," was authored by the AAP Task Force on the Promotion of Breastfeeding and published in 1982. The second statement, titled "Breastfeeding and the Use of Human Milk," was authored by the AAP Work Group on Breastfeeding and published in 1997. The third statement, also titled "Breastfeeding and the Use of Human Milk," was authored by the AAP Section on Breastfeeding and published in 2005. As AAP's most recent statement on infant feeding, the 2005 document still stands as the organization's official statement of policy. Whereas the 1982 statement reinforced the topos of breastfeeding as foundation, the latter two statements have served as pronouncements of the organization's new stance on infant feeding, which can be described in terms of the topos of breastfeeding as the norm. Although chronological order demands that we begin by examining the 1982 policy statement, our most important purpose, as we shall see, is to expose the rhetorical work that has been necessary to accomplish the significant changes that are reflected in the 1997 and 2005 policy statements.

Insofar as they recommend specific evidence-based guidelines for clinical practice, these infant-feeding policy statements bear some resemblance to the charter documents that communication researchers have previously studied. Such documents include the *Diagnostic and Statistical Manual of Mental Disorders* in psychiatry and the Standard of Care documents that aim to standardize treatments by providing national guidelines specific to each known type of cancer.[1] In medical settings, such documents "serve as the means by which discussions among medical professionals take place and a greater understanding of disease and treatment plans are constructed."[2] However, these infant-feeding policy documents are not, strictly speaking, intended as clinical guidelines in the same manner as the charter documents that have been studied by previous communication scholars. One important difference is that these AAP policy statements on infant feeding have attained a high public profile, something that was considered important to those who drafted the documents. Dr. Lawrence Gartner emphasizes that AAP policy statements are highly visible in various segments of the public sphere beyond the pediatrics community:

> "I think [AAP] statements have gained a great deal of respect and that's true not just for the public in general. . . . Public health people, federal agencies like Health and Human Services . . . feel very strongly that the Academy of Pediatrics must be consulted on all issues related to child health, and I think that they are looking for help from us. . . . I think the impact of whatever the Academy says is enormous, which also puts a considerable responsibility on to all of us . . . who write these things, to be sure that what we're saying is valid, documented." (telephone interview, November 13, 2000)

Thus, unlike the charter documents analyzed in previous communication research, most of which were written exclusively for audiences of scientific and medical experts, the three AAP statements on infant feeding were written for much broader audiences, including medical experts and also parents, public-health authorities, policy makers, and the media. As Gartner suggested, AAP policy statements recommend specific medical practices supported by scientific evidence, but they must present such recommendations in language that is accessible and persuasive to broader audiences outside the medical community.

To explain this complex rhetorical function and to illuminate the role that AAP policy statements have played in effecting change in infant-feeding policy and practice, the rhetorical concept of articulation is useful.[3] As it is used here, articulation means a relationship or connection between disparate elements when the relationship becomes naturalized or starts to seem like a reflection of an underlying order. Along these lines, articulation is defined by Stuart Hall as "a linkage which is not necessary, determined, absolute and essential for all time."[4] In such a conceptual relationship, according to Hall, "the two parts are connected to each other, but through a specific linkage that can be broken." As Hall goes on to explain: "You have to ask, under what circumstances can a connection be forged or made? So the so-called 'unity' of a discourse is really the articulation of different, distinct elements which can be re-articulated in different ways because they have no necessary belongingness."[5]

This concept of articulation is useful for the insights that it offers on the rhetorical function of policy documents such as the ones that the AAP has published on infant feeding during the last few decades. If we rely on commonsense understandings of these policy documents' rhetorical function, we might assume that the statements simply transmit or translate preexisting expert information and that the goal of such documents is to achieve symmetry between the sender and receiver of a message: even if the intended receiver of a message does not initially possess the same specialized expertise as the sender, the goal is to design a message that transmits or translates technical information to a nonexpert audience (or possibly an audience who possesses expertise in a different area) in such a way that the same fundamental meaning is maintained when the knowledge moves from sender to receiver.[6] By contrast, when we think in terms of articulation, the relationships among technical documents, the subject matter they convey, and the contexts in which they are situated are seen as complex and dynamic from the outset. Reflecting these ideas, Jennifer D. Slack, David J. Miller, and Jeffrey Doak define articulation as "a particular connection of elements that, like a string of connotations, works to forge an identity that can and does change." Such identities are defined quite loosely: they "might be a subject, a social practice, an ideological position, a discursive statement, or a social group."[7] Thus, thinking in terms of articulation, when expert information is communicated in a technical document, there is no guarantee, even in an optimal situation, that the result will be symmetry between sender and receiver; in fact, there is no guarantee that the identity of sender and receiver will remain the same throughout the process of message transfer. Rather, the communicative act must be seen as situated in a complex network of power and ideological influence. That network is constantly in flux, subject to change, and thus the persuasive technical document is one that makes new meanings, forges new identities, and redraws the lines of ideological influence in a manner that helps to advance the goals of the organizations, groups, or individuals defined as its authors. A key element of this larger reconfiguration, and one that takes on particular importance in the controversies that surround infant-feeding policy, is a continual flux and instability in the relationship between the scientific knowledge and clinical recommendations on infant feeding, even though each policy document depicts science as the motivating force and stable reality behind its policy recommendations.

Applying this concept of articulation to the context of infant-feeding policy, then, we can understand that policy documents such as those published by the AAP do much more than just neutrally transmit or translate knowledge across the boundaries that separate the policy makers, health-care professionals, and others who possess varying types of expertise relevant to infant feeding.

Rather, as the documents communicate such knowledge, they also articulate identities that might appear to be perfectly natural, including the identities of those people or groups who constitute the intended audiences for infant-feeding policy documents and even the identities of those who author such official documents. Perhaps most important is that the three AAP policy documents forge new articulations between the scientific research and the clinical recommendations that pertain to infant feeding. By understanding the science-medicine relationship as an articulation, we start to see how much rhetorical work can be necessary to produce the appearance of an uncomplicated, inevitable relationship between what is known in the context of scientific research and what is advised in the context of clinical practice.

The 1982 Policy Statement

As we have seen, much of the twentieth-century rhetorical history of infant-feeding policy in the AAP has played out against the backdrop of the topos of breastfeeding as foundation. In practical terms, this situation has meant that health-care professionals have tended to treat bottle-feeding as the norm in medical practice even though official medical discourse has supported breast-feeding as the foundation for successful infant feeding. Often with reference to the explosion of knowledge about human milk's role in the immune system that had developed within the past few decades, several publications in the 1970s and early 1980s began to break with this long-standing tendency to treat breastfeeding as merely a foundation. Some of these publications contain scathing criticisms of pediatricians' relaxed approach to the breast–bottle decision. For instance, drawing an analogy between formula use for human infants and several failed attempts to use artificial feeding substances in livestock populations, John W. Gerrard argued in 1974 that "the scientist usually endeavors to make sure that a projected new form of treatment is tried out initially on an experimental animal. In the matter of infant feeding, the experiment, which is artificial feeding, was carried out first in human beings. It was thought to have been successful. Its unsuccessful application in the pig and calf suggests that it was not. We are now beginning to realize, hopefully before it is too late, that there is no adequate substitute for breast milk."[8]

Other authors adopted a more reserved scientific tone. For instance, a 1978 commentary stated that "breast-feeding is strongly recommended for full-term infants, except in the few instances where specific contraindications exist. Ideally, breast milk should be practically the only source of nutrients for the first four to six months for most infants."[9] A 1980 commentary reiterated this idea: "the benefits [of breastfeeding] to the neonate and the mother are so numerous that pediatricians should strongly encourage the practice."[10]

The conflict between this burgeoning support for breastfeeding and those in the pediatrics community who were not interested in changing deeply entrenched practices came to a head in a heated debate that unfolded in the commentaries and letters to the editor sections of the September 1981 and February 1982 issues of *Pediatrics* (just prior to the first AAP policy statement, which appeared in May 1982). The debate in *Pediatrics* was sparked by the AAP's 1981 decision not to endorse the World Health Organization Code of Marketing Breastmilk Substitutes, which aimed to reverse the worldwide decline in breastfeeding rates by restricting the marketing practices of formula manufacturers. Defenders of this AAP decision argued that there was not enough scientific evidence to prove that formula-marketing practices had contributed to the decline in breastfeeding. They emphasized the complexity of assigning blame for this decline, and they argued that to blame formula manufacturers was to oversimplify a complex situation. For instance, in a 1981 commentary that defended the AAP decision, Charles D. May wrote the following: "The crucial point for pediatricians to realize is that during more than five years of debate and hearings, no substantial, sound, scientific data were ever set forth by the critics of industry or officials of the WHO to support the claim that marketing practices for infant formulas have actually been a significant factor in decline in prevalence of breastfeeding in the Third World or anywhere else."[11]

Supporters of the AAP decision also expressed concern that marketing restrictions would impede free enterprise. By contrast, critics of the AAP's decision argued that, even in the absence of clear scientific evidence, the AAP was ethically obligated to join the worldwide activist effort to restrict formula manufacturers' marketing practices. These critics contended that such obligations outweighed any concerns about free enterprise.

In the context of this ongoing debate within the AAP, the ostensible reason for publishing the 1982 AAP policy statement, "The Promotion of Breastfeeding," was to report the results of a study that had just been conducted by the AAP Task Force on the Promotion of Breast Feeding. The stated aim of that study was to explore how mothers' infant-feeding choices were influenced by various factors, including formula-marketing practices as well as other variables. It is interesting to note that the language in the 1982 statement downplayed the controversy surrounding the AAP's decision not to endorse the World Health Organization code. Specifically, the statement claimed that "the Academy endorses the stated aim of this Code," but it went on to justify the academy's decision not to endorse the code (without referring explicitly to that decision).[12] To accomplish these rhetorical goals, the statement authors emphasized the code's overly simplistic approach "to an issue that is complex and involves extensive social, economic, and motivational factors."[13]

In the statement's emphasis on the recent scientific study as the exigency that led to the policy statement, and the concomitant downplaying of the WHO controversy, we begin to see how a technical document can forge an articulation between a particular body of scientific knowledge about infant feeding and a particular set of clinical recommendations on infant feeding. In this case, by foregrounding the recent study as the occasion that led to the statement, the document presented a simple, clean view of a quite complex rhetorical situation. It is easy to look back from today's perspective and determine that various factors led to the need for this policy statement to be published at this time—as is the case with any rhetorical exigency, it was complicated, and many different factors contributed to the need for this statement. Acknowledging some of this complexity might have entailed citing different bodies of scientific evidence, which might have led in turn to different types of clinical recommendations. But by foregrounding the findings of this particular study on marketing practices as the primary reason why the policy statement needed to be written and published at that time, this document downplayed the significance of other complicating factors and perpetuated the impression of a straightforward, inevitable relationship between what was known in the context of scientific research on infant feeding and what was advised in the context of clinical practice.

In articulating the rhetorical situation or exigency that ostensibly required the AAP to publish a policy statement, the 1982 document also delineated how its audience would be configured for years to come. In particular, the 1982 document perpetuated a rhetorical situation in which the formula industry (and those in the medical community who had close ties with this industry) would continue to be the segment of its audience that was most important to please. In so doing, the policy statement authors granted this segment of their total audience more power than the other competing segments. The language that the authors chose seemed to be the most prudent way to address the complex rhetorical situation that they faced. But this language also to some extent shaped what we currently know about that situation by providing the official record now used to understand that moment in history. On the one hand, it seems, the pediatrics community was increasingly under pressure to take a stronger stance in support of breastfeeding. On the other hand, there was a powerful contingent within the pediatrics community who did not want to jeopardize the long-standing relationship between pediatricians and formula companies. The 1982 statement's language suggests an effort to negotiate this delicate balance by downplaying the AAP's recent decision not to endorse the WHO code and advising pediatricians to continue the long-standing practice of treating human milk and formula as relatively equal.

We might say that the 1982 policy statement articulated the existence of its own audience. This rhetorical move is evident in the way that the 1982 statement addressed and represented the formula industry as both a segment of its audience and as a key player in the ongoing rhetorical situation that surrounded infant feeding in the early 1980s. For instance, in presenting the results of its recent study, the policy statement interpreted those results to indicate that formula-marketing practices should not be exclusively blamed for the decline in breastfeeding: "Any discussion of the incentives or deterrents to breast-feeding must focus on the factors surrounding the decision about how the infant is to be fed. This issue is so complex that it is difficult to study in a controlled fashion; but the greater potential for harm comes from ignoring the complexity and focusing on a single variable as the all important determinant."[14] As further evidence to support their contention that formula-marketing practices should not be physicians' primary target, the authors stipulated that the early twentieth-century decline in breastfeeding "began to occur before the present infant formula industry was well developed" and that "the renewal of breast-feeding has taken place at a time when the formula industry is highly developed and its promotion is active."[15]

After addressing the numerous factors, other than formula advertising, that influence mothers' infant-feeding choices, the remainder of the document outlined the history of U.S. infant-feeding practices and emphasized the ways in which medicine's affiliation with the formula industry had presumably benefited the general public. As part of this historical discussion, the 1982 statement referred explicitly to some of the other pro-breastfeeding texts that the AAP published in the years just prior to 1982. It acknowledged these texts and then quickly moved on, presenting its own recommendations as if they were intended to build on these earlier documents' ideas, even though the 1982 statement's recommendations were actually much more neutral (and formula-friendly) than the pro-breastfeeding ideas expressed in some of the statements to which it referred. In fact, even though the 1982 document was titled "The Promotion of Breastfeeding," its statements about the benefits of breastfeeding were not prominent because they were carefully embedded within this carefully orchestrated historical narrative. The following paragraph is indicative of how the document treated breastfeeding promotion: "From a historic and scientific perspective much effort has gone into the development of breast milk substitutes. Pediatricians and the academy have played a key role in ensuring the safety and nutritive quality of alternative methods of infant feeding. Given this history, it is entirely appropriate and significant now that we reemphasize the superiority of breast-feeding."[16]

The authors of the 1982 statement also used language that modified the academy's encouragement of breastfeeding by stipulating that physicians should avoid making mothers feel guilty: "Educational materials should be factual and designed to present the advantages of breast-feeding but should not promote guilt among non-breast-feeding families."[17] Although the "Conclusions" section of the document reiterated "the superiority of human milk," it also stip-ulated that infant feeding is ultimately a matter of choice: "A woman should have the opportunity prior to the time of delivery to make a fully informed decision to breast-feed or not to breast-feed her infant."[18] Along these lines, the "Recommendations" section of the document made clear that informing parents about what kind of breast-milk substitutes should be used is just as important as promoting breastfeeding: "Pediatricians should work to improve the knowledge of all potential expectant and current parents on optimal infant nutrition, emphasizing the positive aspects of breast-feeding and the proper choice and utilization of breast milk substitutes."[19] In short, the language of the 1982 statement seems carefully crafted to express the academy's general support of breastfeeding, but to do so in a way that would not draw too much attention to the uniqueness of human milk or distinguish it too sharply from formula.

Thus, in retrospect it seems that the 1982 document's purpose was not to recommend any changes in infant-feeding practices but to ensure that official AAP policy would reflect the same practices that pediatricians had gener-ally been using for the last several decades. These long-standing practices included treating human milk and formula as interchangeable substitutes and treating the formula industry as an important stakeholder in infant-feeding policy by using language that was certain not to offend industry representa-tives. This attempt to enforce the status quo was particularly important at the time because, as noted above, other ideas about infant feeding were begin-ning to produce vigorous debate and conflict in the pediatrics community just prior to the publication of the 1982 statement. In other words, even though it reported the results of a recent scientific study, the actual rhetorical purpose of the 1982 document was to articulate a particular rhetorical situation and audi-ence identity, not just to communicate the new truths and ideas that appear as its ostensible exigency. By foregrounding the results of the recent study in this manner, the document told readers what the exigency was for the document. More important, the statement defined that exigency in a particular way and highlighted one specific element of this exigency (the study that was recently conducted) rather than emphasizing various other elements of the exigency that also existed at the time. In so doing, this document also worked to stabilize the power relations that had long prevailed among various segments of its audience; that is, it helped to reinforce a status quo in which the interests of formula-industry representatives were closely intertwined with those of the AAP.

From 1982 to 1997

The 1997 policy statement attained a high profile in the medical commu-nity and in the mass media because it urged women to breastfeed for at least the first year of the infant's life. More important, as we have seen, the 1997 statement stipulated that breastfeeding is "the reference or normative model against which all alternative feeding methods must be measured with regard to growth, health, development, and all other short- and long-term outcomes."[20] In contrast to the 1982 statement's careful efforts to balance breastfeeding promotion with approval of bottle-feeding, the 1997 statement offers specific advice to govern physicians' and mothers' interpretations of the breastfeeding body—advice intended to reassure them in the face of infant behavior that might seem worrisome in a culture accustomed to bottle-fed babies. For instance, the statement affirms that it is normal for breastfed babies to eat frequently, advising mothers to allow their babies to eat "whenever they show signs of hunger" rather than try to adhere to a rigid feeding schedule, and it spells out what health-care practitioners should expect to see in the normal nursing mother–baby pair.[21]

The exigency that prompted the 1997 statement, according to its abstract, was "the considerable advances that have occurred in recent years in the scientific knowledge of the benefits of breastfeeding, inthe mechanisms underlying these benefits, and in the practice of breastfeeding." The rhetorical aim of the statement, as also stated in the abstract, is to summarize "the benefits of breastfeeding to the infant, the mother, and the nation, and [set] forth principles to guide the pediatrician and other health care providers in the initiation and maintenance of breastfeeding."[22] Thus, similar to the 1982 statement, this 1997 policy statement uses language that emphasizes new scientific evidence as the exigency that prompted its publication. But also, as was true of the 1982 statement, the rhetorical exigency for the statement was actually far more complex than this emphasis on new scientific evidence might seem to imply. The 1997 policy statement represents the work of a coalition within AAP that emerged in the early 1990s and was solidified in 1994 when the Work Group on Breastfeeding was established. According to Dr. Lawrence Gartner, who chaired the committee responsible for writing the 1997 statement, this document "wasn't written out of a vacuum" (telephone interview, November 13, 2000). Although there were people in the academy concerned about breastfeeding and urging the academy to reject the formula-friendly stance conveyed in the 1982 statement, Gartner explained that these people did not form an active coalition until the Work Group on Breastfeeding was established:

> "I went to the academy and said, you have [breastfeeding] experts here in the academy. . . . You have to pull them together into a group that can really be effective. And they accepted that and said OK, we'll create this work group. . . . There were people . . . who were out there doing stuff, but none of us was sitting around the same table, working together to create documents or recommendations or to teach. But now we're pulled together

into a single structure, I think we're a strong organization within the academy." (telephone interview, November 13, 2000)

In addition to illuminating how the 1997 statement articulated the document's exigency, Gartner's comments illustrate how the authorship of any particular document is not a given, stable identity that automatically preexists the drafting of the document. Rather, the identity of a document's author (or authors) in itself comes to exist through rhetorical acts such as those that culminated in the AAP's adoption of the 1997 statement. As explained by Slack, Miller, and Doak, "any identity," including that of a document's author, "is culturally agreed on or, more accurately, struggled over in ongoing processes of disarticulation and rearticulation."[23] Thus, even though the 1982 and 1997 statements were both officially authored by the AAP, different authorial identities are articulated in each statement. The authorship of the two documents was to some extent mediated by the changes in rhetorical situation that occurred from 1982 to 1997. In fact, in the 1997 document one might say that establishing a new group of authors—that is, people with the authority to draft a solidly pro-breastfeeding statement—was actually a large part of the rhetorical activity that had to take place for the document to be created.

Establishing that group of experts, and having the organization recognize them as experts on breastfeeding, were prerequisites for drafting a new policy statement that would replace the 1982 document. But even though the work group was charged with drafting a new policy statement, the content they would generate for that statement was not necessarily new to them; rather, the statement seemed to crystallize a set of ideas and knowledge that had been circulating for a long time prior to that statement's publication. In fact, as discussed above, a handful of AAP publications in the 1970s and 80s had already taken a stronger pro-breastfeeding stance than that which was adopted in 1982.[24] These earlier documents had proclaimed that breastfeeding offers unique health benefits and that mothers should know these benefits. In such publications, the emphasis on promoting breastfeeding was accompanied by an often repeated list of recommendations aimed at making hospital practices more conducive to breastfeeding: encouragement of rooming-in, efforts to make staff more knowledgeable supporters of breastfeeding, and discouragement of supplementation, to name a few. Many of these recommendations were similar to the ones that were ultimately included in the final version of the 1997 policy statement. A 1981 *Pediatrics* article written by the AAP Committee on Nutrition even anticipated the stance that would eventually be adopted in 1997 by using the term *normal* to describe breastfeeding: "The unique biologic advantages of human milk justify the promotion of lactation as the normal method of infant feeding."[25] Thus, the 1997 statement's recommendations were not necessarily as new as we might be led to believe by its language.

However, none of these earlier documents was an official policy statement, and, therefore, none had been able to achieve the same level of influence as the 1997 statement.

Considered in the context of the discursive struggles occurring from the 1970s to the time it was published, the 1997 statement represented a rhetorical victory for those who had long pushed the pediatrics community to loosen its ties with the formula industry and pronounce a stronger pro-breastfeeding stance. It is important to acknowledge, though, that this victory was not easy. As Gartner describes the situation that has surrounded both of the pro-breastfeeding policy statements (including the 1997 statement and also the 2005 revision of that statement):

> "Yes, the Academy is really strict about this. Any section that has any, or any committee that has any interest in a particular area gets to review the policy statement and critique it. And they also often have outside people who are not in the academy, other organizations or investigators whom we ask to look at documents. So it does go through a very thorough review process. Even before it gets to that, the breastfeeding policy statement took us, I guess each time we did it, it took two years or more of actual work going back and forth within the committee itself, adding things, adding references, revising wording and so forth. It's quite time consuming." (telephone interview, April 28, 2008)

Gartner's words echo our earlier conclusion that there was never a moment when the scientific evidence jumped out and spoke so clearly as to produce an instant consensus among medical experts. Rather, individuals passionately devoted to the cause of breastfeeding advocacy and well versed in the science behind it have had to fight at every step of the way to make the case that human milk has unique properties not available in formula. In the decade and a half that separated the 1982 and 1997 statements, these breastfeeding advocates were fighting on several fronts. One of their most important rhetorical struggles, according to the minutes from several meetings that took place in the years leading up to the 1997 statement, was their engagement in ongoing disputes about the AAP's stance on various international initiatives aimed at curtailing formula-industry influence in hopes of increasing overall breastfeeding rates.

As noted above, the 1982 policy statement was written at a time of great confusion about the AAP's position on the WHO Code of Marketing of Breast Milk Substitutes. By 1994, when the Work Group on Breastfeeding was formed, that controversy seemed to have subsided, but it was being replaced by another similar controversy arising from questions about U.S. involvement in (and potential AAP endorsement of) UNICEF's Baby-Friendly Hospital Initiative (BFHI). In fact, one of the items in the document that officially stated the charge of the Work Group on Breastfeeding when it was initially formed was to review the "Ten Steps for Successful Breast-feeding" as revised by the Expert Work Group of the BFHI and determine whether the academy should endorse this document.

The BFHI involved a series of breastfeeding-friendly practices that hospitals could adopt and then, subject to a successful inspection, receive the BFHI certification. This was a complex discussion, but the most important stumbling block in the situation seemed to have been that U.S. hospitals were unwilling to give up free formula samples, and UNICEF was unwilling to compromise on this issue. Thus, for instance, a letter written by J. P. Grant on behalf of UNICEF to the Expert Work Group charged with investigating the feasibility of U.S. involvement in this initiative included the following language:

> It may be argued that this standard [the requirement to refuse free and low-cost formula products] is too strict for the United States. It is probable that only a handful of hospitals would now meet the Baby-Friendly Hospital Initiative (BFHI) criteria as currently implemented around the world simply because so few U.S. hospitals pay for formula. Let me, however, stress that the dual stipulations that a hospital follows the Ten Steps and refuses any free or low-cost supplies are an absolute prerequisite to receiving global recognition. It is much more important to UNICEF that the integrity of the global initiative be maintained than that a large number of U.S. hospitals receive recognition. The BFHI is best as a standard of excellence in breastfeeding policies and practices rather than as a "least common denominator" that most can attain without considerable commitment.[26]

When this letter was written, the Work Group on Breastfeeding had not yet been officially established. Thus, the entities in AAP that were assigned to deal with the issues surrounding BFHI were the Committee on Community Health Services and the Council on Pediatric Practice. On June 13, 1994, a letter from Joe M. Sanders, AAP executive director, communicated that the AAP, based on these two committees' recommendations, had decided not to endorse the latest version of the BFHI. Sanders's letter suggests that the remaining issues that surrounded the question of AAP endorsement of the BFHI were one of the main justifications for forming a work group on breastfeeding. Specifically, his letter said: "In order to address the concerns that the Academy leadership has with the Ten Steps, the AAP Board of Directors has decided to convene a Work Group on Breast-feeding. Comprised of pediatricians who are experts in the field, the Academy will look to members of the Work Group for advice on how to proceed with several breast-feeding related issues, including Academy endorsement of the Ten Steps document."[27] It is interesting that at its first meeting on July 18, 1994, the AAP Work Group on Breastfeeding upheld the earlier AAP decision not to endorse the BFHI. The reasons recorded in the meeting minutes to support this decision indicate that the work group felt the guidelines for U.S. hospitals, which constituted the particular document they were being asked to endorse, had been watered down too much from the original UNICEF intentions.

Again, the sticking point in the work group's deliberations seemed to be U.S. hospitals' acceptance of free formula. As noted in the meeting minutes: "This new version has at least one additional item added which was not in the previous version. This item concerns a recommendation for review by hospitals of the impact of their accepting free or low cost infant formula. It was noted that the original recommendation of UNICEF indicated that hospitals not accept free or low cost formula. UNICEF continues to insist that the refusal by hospitals to accept free and low cost formula is an essential component of the global Baby Friendly Hospital Initiative."[28]

Because they felt the guidelines had been so weakened from the original global version, then, the Work Group on Breastfeeding recommended that the AAP support the intent and concept of UNICEF's BFHI and remain supportive of efforts to improve the ability of hospitals to increase the incidence of breastfeeding, but that it not endorse the Healthy Mothers / Healthy Babies Coalition Baby-Friendly Hospital Initiative Feasibility Study Expert Work Group document entitled the "US Breastfeeding Health Initiative" of May 1994.[29]

This behind-the-scenes rhetorical activity serves as another example to illustrate how closely intertwined were the interests of the U.S. formula industry and certain segments of the medical establishment in the years leading up to the 1997 statement. It is equally important to note, however, that the medical establishment itself, even within the confines of the AAP, was deeply conflicted on this issue. This series of events serves to illustrate one important message: that loosening the ties that held together this long-standing articulation between the formula industry and the medical establishment were important rhetorical goals of the 1997 statement. Weakening this articulation ultimately effected fundamental changes in the configuration of the audiences for AAP policy statements and in the larger rhetorical situation that surrounded such statements.

Meeting minutes and other documents from the years that preceded the 1997 statement suggest that the work group felt it was becoming increasingly important for the AAP to express a consistent stance on breastfeeding amid all the confusion that had surrounded the organization's stance on recent global initiatives. For instance, an "Intent for Statement" document dated September 20, 1994, described the policy statement that the work group planned to write as follows: "A new comprehensive policy statement on breastfeeding would give the Academy a cohesive, consistent position on breastfeeding. This is necessary as there are a number of other statements and components of Academy publications which are not in complete agreement with each other."[30]

Reflecting another important theme, some documents suggest that "science" was perceived as the key to achieving the more consistent stance desired. For instance, a document titled "Intent for Subject Review" stated the following: "In the past few decades, the information available about the benefits of breast-feeding and the value of human milk has changed significantly. The 'science' of breast-feeding is often overlooked as physicians try to support exhausted, busy young mothers in their attempts to breast-feed. This scientific documentation of the value of breast-feeding and human milk will provide state-of-the art information for mothers in their decision to breast-feed."[31]

Such language reinforces the idea that the scientific knowledge and clinical recommendations on infant feeding do not exist in an inevitable, natural relationship to each other but rather in an articulation that is constantly subject to renegotiation. Such language also suggests that, just as in the case of the 1982 statement, it was a complex rhetorical situation that preceded the 1997 statement. The formula industry was an important, if seemingly silent, player in the controversy. Although formula representatives were not necessarily sitting at the tables where AAP infant-feeding policy was made (to the best of my knowledge), they exerted influence on the larger rhetorical situation in which infant-feeding policy was made by giving free formula samples that hospitals did not want to give up.

Meeting minutes and other documents suggest that in the years leading up to the 1997 statement, and especially before the Work Group on Breastfeeding was formed in 1994, a great deal of confusion and uncertainty about the AAP stance on infant feeding existed within the organization—so much confusion and uncertainty that it is probably not accurate to think of this organization as a unified entity with regard to infant-feeding policy in the years preceding the 1997 policy statement. As is often the case when an official policy statement of any kind is drafted in a large organization, managing this confusion and uncertainty appears to have been one of the most important challenges faced by the newly formed work group that was charged with authoring the 1997 AAP policy statement.[32] "Science" seemed to figure as the potential mediator of this conflict-ridden rhetorical situation.

This emphasis on science as the exigency for the statement persisted in the language that appeared in the final version of the 1997 statement. Although pediatricians have always believed breastfeeding to be optimal, the statement suggests, researchers had recently discovered scientific evidence of the benefits of human milk more compelling than that available before: "Extensive research, especially in recent years, documents diverse and compelling advantages to infants, mothers, families, and society from breastfeeding and the use of human milk for infant feeding."[33] This new evidence, according to the 1997 statement, had led to a new certainty that breastfeeding is not only optimal, as suggested in the 1982 statement, but that it is the norm.

As examples of the "considerable advances that have occurred in recent years," the statement cites a total of fifty-two studies on its first page. Thirty-seven of these are epidemiologic studies demonstrating human milk's protection against disease in the infant; of the remaining fifteen studies, two pertained to the infant's cognitive development, nine to health benefits for breastfeeding mothers, and four to the social and economic benefits of breastfeeding. Thus, the statement presents its new recommendations primarily as a response to new epidemiologic evidence. Clearly, then, scientific evidence did play an important part in the ability of the Work Group on Breastfeeding to make a successful argument, as was anticipated in the archival documents that record discussions leading up to the drafting of the statement. However, what might not be apparent in either the meeting minutes or the final version of the policy statement is that the rhetorical situation at that time demanded not just any "science," but rather a quite specific type of scientific evidence: the statement authors needed scientific evidence that would make beliefs about human milk's immune-protective qualities convincing enough to a wide enough group of people that such evidence would be seen as the logical basis for AAP infant-feeding policy.

Such evidence became available in a group of 1990s studies suggesting that the immune protection human milk afforded was significant in all socio-economic groups, even in developed countries. Previous studies had not been able to establish this widespread significance. Thus, it is important that the 1997 statement was able to state that current research in "developed countries, among predominantly middle-class populations" proves the importance of human milk's immune protection.[34] As this sentence indicates, previous scientific evidence had demonstrated the existence of antibodies in human milk, and it had demonstrated the significance of this protection in some populations, but it had not entirely convinced a sufficiently wide segment of stakeholders in infant-feeding policy that human milk's immune protection was necessary in developed countries and middle-class populations. Skeptics (or those who would defend the long-standing alliance between medicine and the formula industry) could always refute the importance of human milk's immune protection by claiming that such protection was not necessary in developed countries such as the United States. And such refutations did exist. For example, in 1984, the AAP journal *Pediatrics* published an extensive supplement to its regular issue. Titled "Report of the Task Force on the Assessment of the Scientific Evidence Relating to Infant-Feeding Practices and Infant Health," the report concluded that, for the most part, the immune protection offered by human milk was not all that significant in developed countries.[35] Another influential article published in 1986 criticized the methods of previous epidemiologic studies and called into question the necessity of human milk's immune protection in developed countries and affluent populations.[36]

By contrast, scientific evidence that became available in the 1990s was used to support claims for the necessity of human milk's immune-protective benefits, even in developed countries, with greater certainty. These studies, all published in the 1990s, claimed to use more sophisticated methods than those used in any of the previous studies.[37] The authors based their conclusions on larger populations, providing a basis to refute the doubts and uncertainty that had apparently clouded the question of human milk's immune protection for past researchers, including those who had authored the 1984 report. The 1997 policy statement cited the studies that produced this scientific evidence as its primary justification and presented its new recommendations as logical responses to this evidence.

Thus, the "considerable advances" to which the 1997 statement attributed its new recommendations were not exactly new scientific discoveries. Rather, they were discoveries that led to a type of evidence that made human milk's immune protection more convincing to a wider audience of stakeholders involved in infant-feeding policy efforts. The 1997 statement presents the more certain evidence as a prediscursive reality, part of its context, as if its new recommendations were just an inevitable, neutral response to this context. But from a rhetorical perspective, the statement itself actually played an important role in constructing this aspect of its context. Even though scientific evidence was available long before this time, and such evidence was solid enough to convince many pediatricians of the necessity of breastfeeding, the policy statement's 1997 publication marks the moment when a much wider audience came to know and accept that science convincingly supports human milk's immune function.

If the 1997 policy statement achieved a victory, then, it was to forge a new articulation between the science and medicine of infant feeding. In this new articulation, scientific evidence on the health benefits of breastfeeding—immune system benefits most notably—were finally granted a serious presence among all the confounding factors that had been used to justify the far less certain stance announced in the AAP's 1982 statement. When we look closely at the language in the 1997 statement and the precise manner in which it incorporated "new" scientific evidence, we see that material changes in the circumstances surrounding infant-feeding policy did occur between 1982 and 1997. But we also see that the 1997 statement's language played an active role in establishing the meaning that would be ascribed to these material changes in circumstances. The 1997 statement did not just report new scientific findings; it articulated a science–medicine relationship very different from that which had preceded the 1982 statement. To understand the science–medicine relationship depicted in the 1997 statement as an articulation means to view this depiction as the discursive manifestation of one particular moment in a power struggle that preceded the 1997 statement and one that also continued to play out underneath the surface of the consensus and certainty communicated in this document. So again we can understand the new meaning produced by the statement as articulation because it involves rearranging and reconfiguring relationships among various elements of the rhetorical situation.

The rhetorical work of the 1997 statement not only led to different infant-feeding recommendations but also fundamentally reconfigured the entire rhetorical situation in which personal, clinical, and policy decisions about infant feeding would subsequently be made. It is not just the case that the same body of scientific evidence became larger or more convincing. Rather, experts arrived at a new consensus about the type of scientific evidence on which infant-feeding recommendations should be based. For instance, as noted above, the 1997 statement cites thirty-nine studies on human milk's immune protection. By contrast, when it comes time to support its claim about the "social, economic, and environmental benefits" of breastfeeding, the statement cites only four studies. When the 1997 statement mentions social factors at all, it depicts them in simplistic terms and subordinates them to the scientific evidence on immune protection. Specifically, the statement's sixth paragraph addresses the "significant social and economic benefits to the nation, including reduced health care costs and reduced employee absenteeism for care attributable to child illness."[38] Even though this language seems to acknowledge the economic and social factors of infant feeding, the statement's recommendations are ultimately based almost exclusively on scientific evidence of human milk's health benefits, primarily immune-system benefits. Much as the 1982 statement had briefly mentioned some of the scientific evidence on human milk's health benefits, without making any substantial effort to acknowledge this evidence in its policy recommendations, the 1997 statement shifts to an emphasis on such scientific evidence and consequently downplays the social and economic factors that were highlighted in the 1982 document.

By foregrounding biological aspects of breastfeeding and minimizing social aspects, the 1997 statement dramatically transforms experts' understanding of breastfeeding as a practice. In sharp contrast to the 1982 statement, which based its claims almost entirely on citations of research on the social and economic aspects of infant feeding, the assumption in the 1997 statement is that the scientific evidence of breastfeeding's health benefits is so convincing, so certain, that it is not acceptable to leave infant-feeding recommendations vague and subject to the complexities and variation that arise if infant feeding is framed as a matter of individual choice as it was in the 1982 statement. As such, in the 1997 statement breastfeeding is articulated as a fundamentally biological act, one that is supported by the best available scientific evidence—

evidence so strong and convincing that it makes unnecessary or irrelevant any kind of concerns construed as "social" rather than strictly scientific.

This shift in understanding is even apparent in the titles of the two documents. The 1982 statement was titled "The Promotion of Breastfeeding." By contrast, in the 1997 statement the language used to depict the preferred feeding method is expanded to "Breastfeeding and the Use of Human Milk." Although it might seem like a subtle difference, this expansion to include "and the use of human milk" reflects the statement's emphasis on biological aspects of infant feeding and the idea that the scientific components of human milk are more important than the means through which that milk is delivered to the infant.

Thus, the 1997 statement clearly creates new linkages and rearranges elements in the rhetorical situation, creating "different possibilities and practices" as it articulates a particular configuration of the relationship between scientific knowledge and clinical recommendations.[39] Although the 1997 statement certainly, to some extent, translates scientific evidence, when we look inside the science–medicine relationship that seems unproblematic on the document's surface, we see that in this case, medical rhetoric does much more than translate; it articulates a relationship between science and medicine very different from that which had informed previous medical policy.

In other words, we can understand the rhetorical significance of the 1997 policy statement in two ways: both as a reflection of changes that had occurred since 1982 and as an agent in effecting such changes. Bowker and Star refer to such a dual rhetorical function as "convergence," which they define as a "process of mutual constitution" in which "information artifacts . . . undergird social worlds, and social worlds undergird these same information resources."[40] In this understanding, a technical document such as this policy statement is seen as neither a neutral reflection of a reality that precedes it nor as a conglomeration of free-floating signifiers, able single-handedly to construct whatever reality its authors desire.

Perhaps not surprisingly, the language in the final version of the 1997 statement obscures the rhetorical work that was necessary to forge the connection between scientific evidence and medical policy and instead portrays the new recommendations as a simple translation of recent "advances." Essentially, then, the statement presents itself as merely a translation of the latest scientific findings. There is nothing unusual about this rhetorical move in a medical document. However, sometimes rhetorical activity that looks like simple translation on the surface can be revealed as articulation when viewed from a different perspective.[41] To see the science–medicine identity as an articulation means to see that the obscuring accomplished by presenting it as a smooth surface is part of a larger effort rhetorically to construct the situation in which infant-feeding policy is made. Entities such as the science–medicine relationship in this document that appear unproblematic on the surface are revealed to be far less stable when viewed as articulations, not only because they obscure part of the reality they presumably represent but also because they play an active part in constituting that reality.[42]

1997 to 2005: Rhetorical Success, but Also New Challenges

Perhaps not surprising, the 1997 statement was enthusiastically received by breastfeeding advocates. It was seen as a long-awaited official endorsement of breastfeeding by the AAP. For instance, in the words of Sharon, one of my early research participants, the 1997 document was "an amazing statement."[43] Sharon was a lactation consultant who, at the time she was interviewed, was working with both inpatient and outpatient mothers in a large urban hospital. As she went on to explain, "I have made stacks of copies and put them in the resident lounge." Although Sharon acknowledged that the statement's guidelines regarding breastfeeding are not mandates that have to be followed, or even read, by any individual physician, she saw the document as powerful because it "set the record straight" on breastfeeding: "It spells out the benefits, it spells out the parameters of normal breastfeeding, that frequent feeding is normal—that some of the things that are viewed as abnormal by some people who are not familiar with breastfeeding are actually normal. Runny stools are normal. And so they set out the parameters of what's normal with breast-fed babies, what are the benefits, and . . . what do you do when you have a problem."

Similarly, Jackie, a La Leche League leader and another of my early research participants, saw the 1997 statement as a significant step for breastfeeding advocates because "they stopped watering it down. They came out and said, yes, it makes a difference." She also expressed her belief that the statement granted credibility to the mother who chooses to nurse for a year or longer, who is likely to receive criticism not only from physicians but also from friends and family members because such long-term nursing is still extremely rare in the United States:

> "Women can now take this statement to their mothers and say the American Academy of Pediatrics said they should keep nursing him even though he's three months old. They can take it back to their doctor and say, you're saying it doesn't make a difference, but the American Academy of Pediatrics says . . . that breastfeeding should continue for at least twelve months, and for as long after as is mutually desired. . . . So the American Academy of Pediatrics statement probably is the single most important

thing that's happened, probably in the last five to ten years, because it's an official body that said, yes, this is important, yes, this makes a difference."

In short, these women saw the 1997 policy statement as a welcome and long-awaited step that the medical community had taken toward rescuing breast-feeding from a history that had treated it as anything but normal.

These words from research participants reinforce the fact that the 1997 policy statement was rhetorically effective because of the new meanings it artic-ulated and the new rhetorical realities that it made possible, both within the realm of medical practice and for the lived experiences of mothers feeding their babies. They also echo the idea that thinking of persuasion as articulation requires us to think beyond immediate concrete changes in evaluating a docu-ment's rhetorical effectiveness. In particular, articulation entails a particular conception of the power of a document such as these AAP policy statements: "Power is no longer understood as simply the power of a sender over a receiver or as the negotiated symmetry of the sender's or receiver's meanings but as that which draws and redraws the lines of articulation."[44] From the perspective of breastfeeding advocates who had long criticized the AAP for not supporting breastfeeding strongly enough because of ties to the formula industry, the 1997 statement's declaration of breastfeeding as the norm represented a bold step away from the various concerns that had caused the AAP to modify its sup-port of breastfeeding in earlier policy statements. Thus, the statement's rhe-torical purpose involved much more than just communicating "new" scientific evidence—that evidence was pulled together into an argument that had as one of its goals the articulation of breastfeeding advocates as an important element of its audience and a simultaneous downplaying of the formula industry in that audience. The 1997 statement not only invoked breastfeeding supporters such as Sharon as an audience but also provided the information (in an authorita-tive format) that members of this audience needed to solidify their position in the ongoing day-to-day rhetorical struggles they faced.

Following this line of inquiry, and extending it to the realm of public pol-icy beyond the statement itself, one might trace how the 1997 statement has articulated medical policy on breastfeeding to a particular body of scientific evidence in a way that impacts not only clinical practice recommendations but also federal public-health initiatives. For instance, the standards that this statement recommended have been cited in subsequent documents such as the federal government's Healthy People 2010 initiatives, which stipulated target breastfeeding rates that are now used as a nationwide benchmark, and the Center for Disease Control's addition of questions on mothers' infant-feeding methods to the National Immunization Survey.[45] In 2003, when the questions on infant feeding were added, this survey became the federal government's first instrument for systematically gathering infant-feeding data as a way to track progress toward these benchmarks at both the state and national levels. Prior to the addition of these questions to the National Immunization Survey, formula companies' marketing surveys were considered the best available information on U.S. breastfeeding rates. Another highly visible example of a public-health effort that occurred in the wake of the 1997 statement was the National Breastfeeding Awareness Campaign initiated in 2004. As we have seen, the designers of this campaign used new scientific evidence of human milk's health benefits as grounds for the depiction of formula-feeding as risky behavior.[46] These examples of public-health initiatives that were made possible by the new pro-breastfeeding stance articulated in the 1997 statement reflect Bowker and Star's suggestion that the classifications contained in the official documents involved in medical policy serve as "scaffolding" for future work that often includes public-health tasks such as "data collection and validation."[47]

In addition to these various effects in the larger realm of public health, the 1997 statement led to changes in the rhetorical dynamics of infant-feeding policy within the confines of the AAP. Perhaps the most significant change was that on July 1, 2000, the Work Group on Breastfeeding became an official section in the AAP. The justification for this change is described as follows in the document that officially proposed that a section should be established: "The proposal to develop a new Provisional Section on Breastfeeding within the AAP derives from a recommendation of the AAP Board of Directors in recognition of the need for the Academy to have a continuing and stable organizational structure to assist the Academy in its efforts to promote, support, and educate in the field of breastfeeding."[48]

The proposal notes that the work group which had authored the 1997 statement was intended to be temporary, with specific tasks, and it had completed these tasks. After those tasks were completed, the group temporarily became a task force that was still working on several objectives. The major justification for transforming the group into a new section included "the need for an entity to assume responsibility for projects and initiatives developed by the Task Force," among several other reasons listed in the proposal.[49] The need to collaborate with other entities in the AAP and with other organizations such as the American College of Obstetricians and Gynecologists was also emphasized in this proposal.

As this language suggests, the 1997 statement was an important milestone, but it did not represent the end of the breast–bottle controversy within the AAP. One challenge that the statement's authors still faced was continuing demands for more evidence, and more certain evidence, of human milk's health benefits. As Gartner observes, demands for more certain scientific evidence steadily increased in the decade subsequent to the mid-1990s when the 1997 statement had been drafted:

> "Yes, there's definitely been a change. During that period, roughly a ten-year period, that decade, the whole issue of evidence-based medicine came into great prominence, and great importance, and everyone now not only saw the importance of actual research data to support what one is saying but also to grade the quality of the research. . . . There's definitely been a move throughout medicine, not just in pediatrics, and not just in breastfeeding, but worldwide to utilize research for whatever claims one is making, which we've always done, but also to be more critical about the papers that you use and to note which ones are stronger, which ones are weaker." (telephone interview, April 28, 2008)

In addition to these continuing demands for new and stronger evidence, consistency within the AAP continued to be a major concern after the 1997 statement was published. For example, minutes from the December 5–6, 1998, meeting of the Work Group on Breastfeeding mention an AAP publication on premature babies, *Announcing the Early Arrival of Our Baby,* and express the group's concern about the way in which that document depicted breast-feeding.[50]

One important function of the newly established Section on Breastfeed-ing was to provide a permanent structure within the organization to continue the Work Group's efforts to achieve consistency across all AAP publications. In fact, there is a notable change in organizational communication patterns after the 1997 statement: after this statement, the Work Group on Breast-feeding (which became the Section on Breastfeeding in 2000) was increasingly recognized as the authoritative entity within the AAP to which to turn when questions came up about infant feeding. For instance, the minutes for the February 27–28, 1999, meeting of the work group report that the group had to address two different infant-feeding issues that had recently come into public view: a surge in the number of cases of vitamin D deficiency among breastfed babies and formula companies' recent attempts to market docosahexaenoic acid (DHA) supplements for breastfeeding mothers and as additives to their products. On the vitamin D question, even though the deficiency involved just a handful of cases, these cases were receiving a great deal of attention, and the Work Group on Breastfeeding decided at its February 27–28, 1999, meeting "that a literature search was appropriate at this time with future consideration for a joint CON [Committee on Nutrition] / Work Group on Breastfeeding statement on Vitamin D and breastfeeding."[51] On the DHA issue, formula companies were making questionable claims about this new additive. Accord-ing to the meeting minutes, "information was shared among work group members regarding the current state of research on DHA, supplementation of infant formulas, and an infant's ability to synthesize DHA."[52]

Although nothing was resolved at this meeting on the issues of vitamin D supplementation or DHA supplements and additives, the fact that these topics were addressed at the work group's meeting is significant because of the organizational change that it represents. Members of the Work Group on Breastfeeding apparently felt it was important to be proactive in addressing these issues so that they could prevent the spread of misinformation that might lead to public perceptions that human milk was somehow faulty—because of vitamin D deficiency or because it contained lower levels of DHA than the newly enhanced formulas. Picking up again on the notion that the 1997 statement reconfigured the rhetorical situation in which infant-feeding policy would be made, it is not surprising to find that those who were inclined to question the uniqueness of human milk as compared to formula would have to make different kinds of arguments if they wanted to be successful. More important, though, observing what happened when the AAP was confronted with the issues of vitamin D and DHA illustrates a key aspect of the larger reconfiguration of the rhetorical situation that occurred after the 1997 statement was published: that statement seemed to solidify the AAP Work Group on Breastfeeding (later, the Section on Breastfeeding) as the place to turn for medical advice when breastfeeding issues came up. By contrast, as noted earlier, there was previously a great deal of confusion surrounding the organization's stance on infant feeding, largely because there was not a solid entity within the organization to serve as the authority on breastfeeding.

These issues of consistency and other challenges, such as vitamin D and DHA, were some of the factors that led the Section on Breastfeeding to perceive the need for an updated policy statement and ultimately led the academy to publish the revised version in 2005. The need for a revision to the 1997 statement was first mentioned at the October 29–30, 2000, meeting of the Provisional Section on Breastfeeding. Specifically, the minutes include the following language expressing the need for a policy-statement revision: "Additional topics and corresponding research to be explored include type II diabetes, environmental contaminants, hypercalcemia/tetany, increased body weight in formula-fed infants after 4 months of age, cytomegalovirus, areas of needed research (including human milk banks), and recognizing the effects of cultural diversity on breastfeeding attitudes and practices."[53]

Continuing the emphasis on science, the 2005 revision of the policy statement, which retained the title of the 1997 statement, cites "significant advances in science and clinical medicine" that had occurred since 1997 as its exigency. The 2005 document continues the 1997 statement's emphasis on breastfeeding as the norm, but it strengthens the academy's position in this regard by citing research that supported a wider range of benefits to the infant and adding to the 1997 statement's recommendations for increasing breastfeeding rates. As the opening paragraph says, "this revision cites substantial new research on the importance of breastfeeding and sets forth principles to guide pediatricians and other health care professionals in assisting women and children in the initiation and maintenance of breastfeeding."[54] After repeating the 1997 statement's language about breastfeeding as a normative model, the 2005 statement includes a new sentence that cites several studies demonstrating specific health benefits for premature infants: "In addition, human milk-fed premature infants receive significant benefits with respect to host protection and improved developmental outcomes compared with formula-fed premature infants."[55] The 2005 statement mentions the immune protection that human milk provides against many of the same diseases mentioned in the 1997 statement, but it adds "late-onset sepsis in preterm infants"[56] to the list and cites two studies to support this claim. It also includes a new statement about infant mortality: "In addition, postneonatal infant mortality rates in the United States are reduced by 21% in breastfed infants."[57] Similar to the 1997 statement, the 2005 statement uses less certain language in referring to studies that suggest human milk's protection against a list of noninfectious diseases that is quite similar to the list of diseases included in the 1997 statement: "Some studies suggest decreased rates of sudden infant death syndrome in the first year of life and reduction in incidence of insulin-dependent (type 1) and non–insulin-dependent (type 2) diabetes mellitus, lymphoma, leukemia, and Hodgkin disease, overweight and obesity, hypercholesterolemia, and asthma in older children and adults who were breastfed, compared with individuals who were not breastfed."[58]

The 2005 statement does include two sections that were not present in the 1997 statement: "Contraindications to Breastfeeding" and "Conditions that are not Contraindications to Breastfeeding."[59] These two sections cite research that helps to clarify misperceptions that health-care professionals might have about the need to advise certain women not to breastfeed. The 2005 statement also includes some new recommendations for promoting breastfeeding, including more precise guidelines on hospital practices that can foster successful breastfeeding. Most notable among its new recommendations is the 2005 statement's language about duration of breastfeeding. The 1997 statement simply stated: "It is recommended that breastfeeding continue for at least 12 months, and thereafter for as long as mutually desired."[60] The 2005 statement, by contrast, makes a much bolder statement in support of extended breastfeeding: "There is no upper limit to the duration of breastfeeding and no evidence of psychologic or developmental harm from breastfeeding into the third year of life or longer."[61]

In short, the differences between the 2005 and 1997 statements are far less significant than the differences between the 1997 and 1982 statements.

Whereas the 1997 statement forged dramatically different articulations of rhetorical situation, audience, and authorship from those which appeared in the 1982 statement, the 2005 statement is better understood as a reinforcement of the articulations that were forged in the 1997 document. This periodic need for reinforcement of the articulations that policy documents set forth has been suggested in previous research on public-policy reports and their role in organizational and social change.[62] Among these previous studies, Carolyn D. Rude's analysis of public-policy reports on environmental issues is particularly relevant to the rhetorical function of AAP policy statements in the long-term process of change. Rude argues that to understand the rhetorical impact of the report by the Union of Concerned Scientists that she examined, we must look beyond traditional definitions of delivery, which center on issues such as document design and language use as applied in individual documents. In the expanded view of delivery that Rude suggests, "the publication is not an end in itself but a means to an end of change in policy and behavior."[63] In the report she examined, we can understand rhetorical success only if we take a long-term view and see that this report provided the information necessary to form a new coalition that made it possible to pursue the Union of Concerned Scientists' rhetorical goals more effectively than one activist organization could do alone: "The coalition itself represents progress toward goals and an example of the extended sense of delivery. Getting more people involved in carrying the message to ever wider audiences may be part of what we come to understand as delivery. One organization cannot accomplish alone what eight can accomplish together."[64]

Rather than judging the effectiveness of technical documents based on whether they immediately persuade their target audiences to take the desired action, then, if we adopt the long-term view of delivery that Rude suggests, we must look for incremental changes in any element of the rhetorical situation and then track, over time, how such incremental changes can snowball into something larger than the sum of their parts. In the case of AAP infant-feeding policy, we can see evidence of this type of incremental change in the 2005 statement's reinforcement of articulations that were first forged in the 1997 statement and rhetorical activity that preceded it.

As we have seen, the authors of the 1997 document faced the difficult rhetorical task of loosening the long-standing articulation between formula-industry interests and those of the medical community. Once that articulation had been loosened enough to make way for the 1997 statement's bold declaration of breastfeeding as the normal infant-feeding method, it then became possible to establish the Work Group on Breastfeeding as a permanent section in the organization, and then, eventually, it was possible to articulate an even stronger pro-breastfeeding stance in the 2005 policy statement.

Similar to the public-sector documents that Rude and other communication scholars have recently examined, then, the rhetorical impact of the three AAP policy statements is most accurately understood if we think about persuasion as a process of long-term change that unfolds over time. That long-term process of change is often punctuated by high-profile documents, such as the 1997 and 2005 AAP policy statements, and these documents undoubtedly play an important role in effecting change. However, in the series of historical events we have examined, no document has single-handedly effected change overnight. The net effect of these documents over time has been not only to inform their audiences of the latest scientific information on infant feeding, as the language of the documents themselves might suggest, but also, and more important, to punctuate a larger process of organizational and social change that has involved a dramatic reconfiguration of the rhetorical situation in which policy discussions about infant feeding take place. Through this larger process of change, a different group of experts has been authorized to speak about infant feeding, the audiences for such policy documents have changed, and, as a result, the rhetorical situation in which experts craft arguments about "breast or bottle" has fundamentally changed as well.

Articulation, Science, and Medicine in the Kairology of Infant Feeding

An important idea in this book is that science and medicine often seem to be so closely intertwined as to appear one and the same. Such an appearance is reinforced in the narratives of scientific progress that are present in official policy language and in the comments of focus-group participants who emphasized new scientific discoveries about health benefits as the main reason why they wanted to breastfeed. This understanding of the relationship between the scientific knowledge and clinical practices pertaining to infant feeding might be said to reflect the traditional assumption that medicine is merely the "benevolent application" of modern science.[65] It also corresponds with the recent push to strengthen medicine's scientific basis through calls for "evidence-based medicine."[66] However, because an articulation such as that between scientific facts and clinical recommendations is non-necessary and subject to change, it can be taken apart, despite its seemingly smooth surface appearance. This breaking apart of seemingly natural connections is the task of a rhetorical critic—to pull apart the science–medicine articulation, or to ask, in Hall's words, "under what circumstances *can* [this] connection be forged or made?"[67] In fact, as we have seen, the scientific knowledge about and clinical recommendations on infant feeding during the last several decades have been subject to a great deal of conflict. Understanding this conflict, most of which has occurred behind the scenes and is obscured by the smooth surface of policy documents when they appear in final form, reveals how much rhetorical work has to be done to articulate the science of infant feeding to the medicine of infant feeding at any given moment in history.

The three AAP policy statements each appeared at a significant moment in the rhetorical struggles that have led to the recent shift from the topos of breastfeeding as foundation to the topos of breastfeeding as the norm. Consistent with the concept of articulation, each policy statement has not only responded to the significant moment, or rhetorical exigency, at which it was published but also has played an active part in constructing that moment. Examining these three AAP policy statements and the rhetorical activity involved in producing them extends the previous chapter's historical analysis by revealing how scientific belief in human milk's immune-protective qualities has come to influence medical recommendations and other kinds of policy with regard to infant feeding. Such an analysis emphasizes that the increasingly sophisticated scientific understanding of human milk's immune-protective qualities examined above constituted only one part of the rhetorical struggle in which breastfeeding advocates have engaged over the last several decades. As convincing as these scientific findings about immune protection were to certain elements of their immediate audiences, such findings did not automatically lead to new medical policy recommendations. Rather, as we have seen, in order for the AAP to sanction the stronger pro-breastfeeding recommendations that appear in both the 1997 and 2005 policy statements, the relationship between scientific research and clinical recommendations related to infant feeding has had to be entirely reconfigured. That reconfiguration has required rhetorical efforts to make the scientific evidence about human milk's unique health benefits convincing to multiple audiences. Furthermore, these audiences have become increasingly wide and diverse with the appearance of each new policy statement.

As we will see, even though it seems as if the science of breastfeeding—particularly mounting scientific evidence of human milk's unique immune-protective qualities—has gained an increasingly strong foothold in discursive framing of the choice between breast and bottle throughout the last three decades, the terrain is still shifting. As has always been the case, the smooth, stable surface that appears in the final versions of official medical texts masks ongoing rhetorical activity and conflict that continues behind the scenes. In the case of infant feeding, it would seem that breastfeeding has gained ground in the ongoing breast–bottle debate. But this does not mean that formula companies have stopped their own rhetorical efforts; rather, these efforts have been forced to take on different forms, and formula companies have continued to increase the amount of money they spend engaging in this ongoing rhetorical battle.

4

....

Viral Rhetoric

Breast and Bottle in Current Promotional Discourse

A poster published by the American Academy of Pediatrics contains the following text about human milk's immune-protective qualities: "New babies are at risk for many infections. It is important that they receive all recommended immunizations. Breast milk is not only the perfect food, but is loaded with infection-fighting substances that help protect babies right from birth. It even makes some immunizations work better. Breastfeeding truly is 'Baby's First Immunization.'"[1] The top half of this poster (see fig. 1) displays a close-up image of a newborn baby suckling at the breast, and in tiny print at the bottom of the poster are references to two scientific articles on breastfeeding and infant immunity.[2]

The advertising materials developed for the National Breastfeeding Awareness Campaign similarly emphasize the immune-protective qualities of breastfeeding. For example, one poster in this campaign shows a large picture of two dandelion seed heads (bearing an intentional resemblance to a pair of breasts), and the text below says in all caps, "BREASTFEED FOR SIX MONTHS. HELP REDUCE YOUR CHILD'S RISK FOR RESPIRATORY ILLNESSES"[3] (see fig. 2). Other print advertisements in the campaign offer variations on the same theme. For example, another poster shows two otoscopes side by side and says at the bottom "BREASTFEED FOR SIX MONTHS. HELP REDUCE YOUR CHILD'S RISK FOR EAR INFECTIONS" (see fig. 3).[4] The television advertisements in this campaign, as discussed above, take a more dramatic approach, emphasizing not only the health benefits of breastfeeding but also the risks of formula-feeding. For example, these commercials depict pregnant mothers engaging in risky

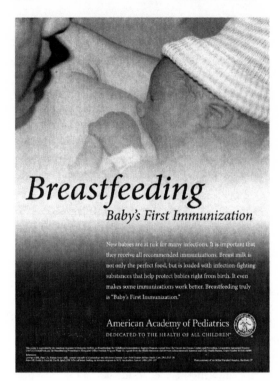

An AAP poster depicts breastfeeding as "baby's first immunization." Fine print at the bottom of the poster cites scientific articles to support this claim. The poster is used with permission of the American Academy of Pediatrics, http://www2.aap.org/ breastfeeding/curriculum/ documents/pdf/BFIZPoster. pdf, copyright American Academy of Pediatrics, 2007.

physical activities such as logrolling and mechanical-bull riding. On-screen text that appears with the visuals says, "You wouldn't take risks before your baby is born . . . Why start after." Finally, a brief voice-over that plays at the end informs listeners that "recent studies show babies who are breastfed are less likely to develop ear infections, respiratory illnesses, and diarrhea. Babies were born to be breastfed."[5] Similar to the AAP poster, then, these advertisements mention specific benefits that all pertain to the immune-protective qualities of human milk.

Many of the messages that are currently being used to promote formula place a similar emphasis on the importance of immune protection and immune-system development to the infant's health. For example, the website of formula manufacturer Similac promotes one of its newer brands of formula, called Similac Advance, by claiming that this product includes an additive called EarlyShield that contains the same immune building blocks as human milk and by describing these newly added elements in scientific terms. Specifically, the website makes the following claims about its latest innovation: "Similac Advance is designed to be more like breast milk and help support your baby's developing immune system. Only EarlyShield has our patented blend of immune-supporting nucleotides—and prebiotics and carotenoids, nutrients naturally found in breast milk. Explore how EarlyShield can help give your baby a strong start."[6] After reading this introductory text, users are repeatedly invited to "learn more" by clicking to navigate through several screens of informational text similar to the excerpt above—text that seems to translate complex scientific information about the infant's immune system in a friendly, easy-to-understand format.

Enfamil currently offers a formula with a "Triple Health Guard" additive that sounds quite similar to Similac's EarlyShield ingredient, although Enfamil's Triple Health Guard includes two other additives besides the prebiotics: one is supposed to produce "healthy growth patterns similar to breastfed babies, in both weight and length" and the other "supports higher mental test scores" and "significantly enhances visual acuity."[7] In promoting this product, the Enfamil website offers the same kind of "learn more" links that Similac offers. The Enfamil site even includes animated visuals to depict the biological events that are supposed to lead to the health benefits offered by each of these three additives.

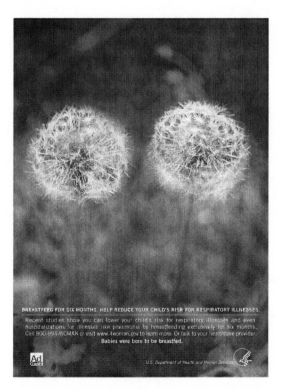

A poster from NBAC urges mothers to breastfeed for six months to "help reduce your child's risk for respiratory illnesses." This poster is available at Office of Women's Health, "Campaign Materials," http://www. womenshealth.gov/ breastfeeding/government-in-action/national-breast feeding-campaign/index. cfm#materials. It is used with permission from the Office of Women's Health.

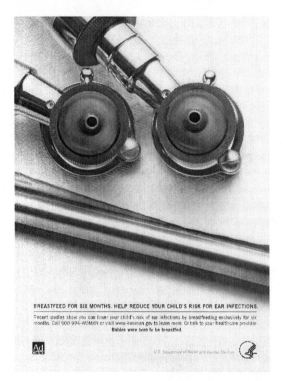

A poster from NBAC urges mothers to breastfeed for six months to "help reduce your child's risk for ear infections." This poster is available at Office of Women's Health, "Campaign Materials," http://www.womenshealth.gov/breastfeeding/government-in-action/national-breast feeding-campaign/index. cfm#materials. It is used with permission from the Office of Women's Health.

As these examples suggest, there are some striking similarities between the messages that today's mothers are hearing about breast- and bottle-feeding, even though the consensus of medical experts in recent years has shifted toward a stronger belief in the unique health-providing qualities of human milk. As we shall see, this apparent resemblance between these two types of infant-feeding messages can be explained by understanding today's formula discourse as a "viral rhetoric" that strategically replicates key elements of the pro-breastfeeding discourse.[8] That is, the discourses that formula companies are currently using to promote their products derive from bits and pieces borrowed from the scientific discourse that promotes breastfeeding. Designers of these formula-advertising messages use these elements from breastfeeding discourse to build persuasive claims about their newest products in much the same way that a virus relies on its host cell to replicate itself endlessly.

To understand exactly how formula discourse functions as a viral rhetoric, we need to look past the surface resemblances between breastfeeding and bottle-feeding discourse and more closely examine the ways in which discourses on each side are talking about the immune system. Such an analysis reveals that formula manufacturers' rhetorical strategies enable them to make claims that sound scientific without reporting any actual scientific evidence. This approach is possible because formula discourse plays by different rules than breastfeeding discourse. For historical reasons that we have outlined above, the requirements to provide supporting evidence are much lower for information that is disseminated in formula advertisements than they have ever been for information on breastfeeding. Because the U.S. Food and Drug Administration (FDA) has always regulated formula as a food product, and because new additives to formula are regulated as supplements rather than drugs, the formula companies have only to prove the safety of new additives to their products, not the efficacy. Furthermore, to prove this safety, formula manufacturers are allowed to conduct their own independent research, without monitoring from any external agency, and then to report the results to the FDA. By contrast, scientific claims about human milk's health benefits have been, and still are, subject to constant scrutiny. Ironically, that scrutiny and demand for increasingly certain evidence have only intensified as the amount and quality of scientific evidence in support of breastfeeding have continued to increase.

Viral Rhetorics

Jenny Edbauer uses the concept of viral rhetoric to explain how specific elements of public discourse can be taken up by different communicators and, therefore, caused to circulate in ways that exceed and extend the boundaries of their initial exigencies. Edbauer's analysis explores the specific example of the Keep Austin Weird slogan that was developed by a local marketing company in the Austin, Texas, area to fight against urban sprawl that resulted from the "dot-com boom" that sparked rapid growth of the city in the 1990s. Although the slogan was initially developed by those who wanted to defend the small independent businesses that populated Austin's downtown from the encroachment of larger corporations such as Starbucks, Edbauer's analysis shows, the slogan became so popular and widely circulated that other entities eventually began using and adapting it to meet their own very different needs. For example, the slogan was taken up by a local literacy campaign, Edbauer notes, and it was used to promote the study of liberal arts at the University of Texas. Ironically, in some of the cases Edbauer analyzes, the entities that took up and adapted this slogan were the same large corporations that the slogan was initially developed to protest against. As just one example, Edbauer notes that after Keep Austin Weird became popular, Cingular Wireless started publishing it next to their corporate logo in publications designed for local circulation in the Austin area.[9]

Edbauer's use of the viral rhetoric concept is part of a larger move among rhetorical theorists toward a new understanding of the rather old concept of rhetorical situation. In broad terms, this movement began with an exchange

between Lloyd Bitzer and Richard E. Vatz concerning the question of whether
individual speakers respond to a preexisting rhetorical situation or play an
active role in constructing that situation as they speak.[10] This general discussion has continued and developed in various directions in contemporary rhetorical theory. Barbara Biesecker, for instance, explains that rhetorical theorists
have traditionally conceived audience, speaker, and rhetorical situation as separate entities that preexist a given act of rhetoric. All three elements might be
modified by the act of rhetoric, but they are still left intact as discrete entities.
In other words, a traditional view of persuasion might lead us to believe that
entities such as the audience and author of a document are "already constituted identities whose operations and relations are determined a priori by a
logic that operates quite apart from real historical circumstances."[11] Instead,
Biesecker asserts, we should conceive "the identity of audience as effect-
structure," and, once we do that, "we become obliged to read every 'fixed'
identity as the provisional and practical outcome of a symbolic engagement
between speaker and audience."[12] Along similar lines, but also attempting to
push Biesecker's redefinition of the rhetorical situation even further, Edbauer
suggests that rhetorical theorists should shift "the lines of focus from rhetorical situation to rhetorical ecologies."[13] Expanding this idea, Edbauer proceeds
to assert that "rhetorical situation is better conceptualized as a mixture of
processes and encounters; it should become a verb rather than a fixed noun or
situs," and to explain that "an ecological or affective rhetorical model is one
that reads rhetoric both as a process of distributed emergence and as an ongoing circulation process."[14]

In a rhetorical ecology, entities such as speaker, text, audience, and exigency do not preexist the act of discourse but rather are constituted through
discursive activity. The notion of viral rhetoric emerges from Edbauer's idea
of rhetorical ecologies as an explanation for the ways in which a popular discursive construct such as Keep Austin Weird can circulate through a rhetorical
ecology, endlessly proliferating and mutating, sometimes in highly unpredictable ways. In Edbauer's words:

> A given rhetoric is not contained by the elements that comprise its rhe-
> torical situation (exigence, rhetor, audience, constraints). Rather, a rhetoric
> emerges already infected by the viral intensities that are circulating in the
> social field. Moreover, this same rhetoric will go on to evolve in aparallel
> ways. . . . What is shared between them is not the situation, but certain
> contagions and energy. This does not mean the shared rhetoric repro-
> duces copies or models of "original" situations. . . . Instead, the same
> rhetoric might manage to infect and connect various processes, events, and
> bodies.[15]

It is this concept of endless proliferation of public messages as they circulate in contexts quite different from their place of origin that is most relevant to our analysis of public messages about breast- and bottle-feeding. Although the messages currently circulating about infant feeding are, of course, quite different from the Keep Austin Weird slogan, there are some important similarities with the situation that Edbauer examines. Just as the Keep Austin Weird slogan was an effective rhetorical move later mimicked by entities and organizations who had very different goals from those who coined the phrase, messages conveying scientific facts about human milk's immune-protective properties are being co-opted by formula companies today.

"Breast Is Best":
Duplicate Sources, Same Message

Given the importance of the immune system in current understandings of health, it is probably not a coincidence that stakeholders on both sides of the rhetorical contest between breast and bottle would conceive immunologic benefits as an effective basis for arguments appealing to their target audiences.[16] However, in light of the long history in which breastfeeding advocates have been required to provide increasingly powerful evidence to distinguish breastfeeding from formula, it is surprising that it would be possible for stakeholders on both sides of this controversy to make arguments that sound so similar. Looking more closely at the manner in which discourses on each side invoke science offers a possible explanation for this resemblance in the surface features of the two discourses.

Breastfeeding advocates within the AAP had to provide increasingly certain scientific evidence of a particular nature to convince the AAP to adopt the stronger pro-breastfeeding stance that was first articulated in the 1997 policy statement. Such evidence is cited in both the 1997 and 2005 policy statements, and it is used to justify the increasingly strong pro-breastfeeding stance expressed in these two statements. It is not surprising that scientific evidence would be required in these policy statements, which are published in the AAP's official journal *Pediatrics* and described as representing the organization's official stance on infant feeding. But it is interesting to note that the same type of evidence cited in these policy statements is present in much of the breastfeeding promotion discourse intended for public audiences.

For instance, the AAP poster that describes breastfeeding as "Baby's First Immunization" cites two scientific articles in footnotes at the bottom of the poster. Both of the studies that this poster cites pertain to the immune-system benefits of human milk, and they were both published in peer-reviewed medical journals. The first is a review article on the immune-system benefits of human milk.[17] It provides a thorough explanation of all the basic concepts related to the infant immune system and cites peer-reviewed articles to support everything that is currently known on this subject. Although this peer-reviewed article presents the information in a much more complex manner than the poster, as we might expect, the cited article lends direct scientific support to the poster's claims that breast milk "is loaded with infection-fighting substances that help protect babies right from birth" and "breastfeeding truly is 'Baby's First Immunization.'" The review article cites 188 references altogether. The second research article cited in the poster is a 1989 study of breastfed versus formula-fed infants that aimed to determine if there was a different immune response to vaccinations.[18] The study reported in this article found there was a significant difference in immune response if the shot was given before the baby had reached one month of age, but not after one month. Although the review article cites several studies that demonstrate a much stronger effect than that suggested by this earlier study, the 1989 article claims to be the first to offer any evidence that breastfeeding heightens an infant's response to immunizations. That is probably why the poster cites the 1989 study rather than any of the more recent studies that have shown a stronger effect. Because these citations are provided, careful readers who have questions about the claims being made in the poster can quite easily look up the articles for themselves.

The presence of these scientific citations in documents intended for public, nonexpert audiences is interesting because, in many ways, it goes against expectations for public-health messages of this nature. As suggested by much of the recent literature on popularization of scientific and medical information, this level of transparency is not typically demanded of messages that communicate scientific or medical information to nonexpert audiences. Rather, language for nonexperts usually communicates such information in ways that imply the audience will accept it at face value without any requirement to cite sources or otherwise prove the legitimacy of the information being presented.[19] Because this AAP poster seems to represent an example of discourse that is intended for public consumption, the fact that it provides these citations to viewers is worthy of further investigation.

The AAP poster is not an isolated example; rather, the tendency to provide scientific citations for the pro-breastfeeding messages that are conveyed in such discourse appears to be widespread. For example, the NBAC website includes a page titled titled "Science behind the Campaign," that lists all the references for the scientific studies that support the campaign's messages.[20] Most of the articles cited on this page report results from studies of large populations of breastfed and formula-fed infants, and they attempt to determine the clinical impact of the immune protection offered by human milk in actual infant populations. The references are presented in four categories that represent the main health benefits on which the campaign focused: defense against diarrhea, otitis media, hospitalization for respiratory illness, and obesity.

Scientific information also seems to lend credibility to the messages that are communicated by the formula websites, but in a different manner. For instance, at the Similac site, the persistent user who continues to click on the appropriate links will eventually come to a page titled "EarlyShield for Immune Support." This page then links to brief videos on nucleotides, prebiotics, and carotenoids: the three elements in EarlyShield that are supposed to support healthy immune-system development and functioning.[21] These pages include animated visualizations that depict the innermost workings of the infant's immune system and show how the tiny elements recently added to Similac help that immune system grow and function. Through such rhetorical elements, viewers presumably gain a basic understanding of current scientific understandings of the immune system (an understanding that, by the way, has been achieved through years of scientific research on the immune components of human milk) and the role that Similac's newly added EarlyShield ingredients purportedly play in helping the "immature" immune system of the infant develop. Each video is narrated with simple explanations, in a gentle female voice, that seem to introduce complex scientific topics in terms basic enough for anyone to understand. For example, the video on prebiotics is accompanied by the following voice-over:

> "So, here's what you need to know about prebiotics. You may not realize it, but your baby's digestive tract is full of billions of bacteria. Bacteria usually get a bad rap. But some of these bacteria actually help keep the digestive system healthy.
>
> "Nature figured this out long ago. Breast milk contains special carbohydrates which act as prebiotics, food for the beneficial bacteria, to help them grow and thrive. EarlyShield also has prebiotics, to support digestive health. And since about 70 percent of the immune system is located in the digestive tract, that's great news for you and your baby."[22]

Similar brief videos (less than one minute long) are available for each of the other elements in EarlyShield (nucleotides and careotenoids), each with a similar voice-over providing the scientific explanation. All three videos are visually pleasing, easy to watch, and easy to understand. There is no way, however, for the user to link to published reports of scientific evidence that would support the site's claims about EarlyShield's function or its effectiveness and not a single reference to such information or a clue as to how an interested user might find such reports.

The Enfamil site uses similar strategies, except that this site goes one step beyond Similac's by making repeated claims that the health benefits of its most recent additives are "clinically proven." No matter which link users might click, the claims they will see about the various additives are said to be supported with "clinically proven" research. Text informs site visitors that "emerging science suggests prebiotic may support your baby's developing immune system," and an image just beneath this text illustrates the three additives that supposedly make Enfamil more like human milk than it used to be.[23] The image includes miniscule symbols that indicate footnotes, as if the site visitor who wants to know more could look up a specific scientific study. However, the language that appears in the footnotes does not provide specific citations for scientific research; it only vaguely mentions that "studies" were conducted. And in fact, despite the numerous references to "clinically proven" claims and "emerging science" that appear throughout this site, there are no links to the results of any scientific studies, and there are no citations provided anywhere in case interested users might want to locate such studies on their own. Although this absence of citations is more in line with what we would expect in popular scientific discourse, it provides an interesting contrast to the examples of breastfeeding discourse examined above.

In other words, the formula websites seem to be doing a great job of looking scientific without providing consumers direct access to any actual scientific data. Although the formula sites seem to provide new scientific information, a closer look reveals that they are actually just repeating key parts of the scientific discourse on current understandings of the infant's immune system without citing any actual evidence to support their claims that current brands of formula might possess some of the same immune-protective qualities as human milk. This contrast between breastfeeding and bottle-feeding discourse hints at what I have dubbed the viral nature of the relationship between these two discourses: it is similar to the manner in which viruses reproduce by inserting genetic information into their host cells as a means of literally "fooling" those cells into producing infinite numbers of new virus copies.[24]

As a viral rhetoric, then, formula discourse might be said to replicate key components of pro-breastfeeding discourse—those components pertaining to the immune system in particular—and to use these components toward very different ends from those for which they were initially intended. The specific sense in which formula discourse might be said to constitute a viral rhetoric is explained by Edbauer's use of the concept and is therefore specifically tied to ongoing efforts to theorize more nuanced conceptions of rhetorical situation. Edbauer's viral rhetoric certainly bears some resemblance to the phrase *going viral* that is frequently used in popular discourse to refer to images, videos, or concepts that rapidly proliferate via social media such as Facebook and YouTube. However, these concepts are not exactly the same. When a video or concept is said to go viral, this simply means it has rapidly proliferated in a way that would not have been possible before the advent of social media. A single YouTube video, for instance, might get hundreds of thousands of views in a surprisingly short period of time because viewers use Facebook, Twitter, and other social media to share it with all of the people in their networks, and then those people share it with their networks, and so on. Such a discourse is viral in the sense that its spread is made possible by the hundreds or thousands of individual users who act as "hosts" that literally cause the "virus" to spread by sharing the text, image, or video with the numerous people in their own social networks, who then pass it on again and again, in a potentially infinite process.

What I am saying about formula discourse is something different. Not only do these discourses rapidly proliferate, as might be the case for a YouTube video; the rhetorical success of formula discourse is also dependent on the fact that its designers are able to borrow and adapt key rhetorical elements from breastfeeding discourse, just as a virus depends on genetic material from its host to infect the host and then quickly replicate itself. In other words, it is the message itself that acts and reproduces in a viral manner, not necessarily the audience members who spread it.

This point can be further illustrated by taking a closer look at the technical documents behind the supposed immune-protective elements that formula companies have recently started adding to their products. As of December 30, 2009, the Similac website text was describing these elements as "nondigestible carbohydrates known as human milk oligosaccharides, which can function as prebiotics."[25] The claims that Similac makes about these "prebiotics" and how they are expected to benefit the infant's immune system are consistent with current scientific understanding of one of the elements in human milk that is believed to offer a similar benefit. As we have noted, when antibodies from human milk were first shown to appear in infants' stools, they were referred to as "coproantibodies," which simply means "antibodies in the stool." Current medical literature uses different terminology and offers a more sophisticated understanding of these immune-protective elements that are now understood to pass from human milk into the infant's gut where they provide a form of immune protection. The literature review cited in the AAP poster examined above describes prebiotics as "substances that enhance the growth of probiotics or beneficial microflora."[26] This definition of prebiotics is quite similar to the explanations provided on the formula websites. For instance, the Similac site describes prebiotics as "special carbohydrates that can be naturally found in breast milk" and claims that these elements, when added to infant formula, "help stimulate the growth of beneficial bacteria in baby's digestive tract to help support the developing immune system." The site further explains this immune-protective role as follows:

Because about 70% of the immune system is found in the digestive tract, developing a strong immune system from birth begins with creating a healthy digestive system. Your baby relies on millions of "good" bacteria in the digestive tract to support immune system development. Special carbohydrates (prebiotics) found in breast milk and Similac Advance Early Shield help stimulate the growth of this beneficial bacteria which helps support your baby's developing immune system.[27]

All of this text is consistent with current scientific understandings, and none of it could be described as inaccurately reporting these current understandings. However, it is important to note that the immune-protective function of prebiotics as described in Lawrence and Pane's literature review is far more complex than that which is offered at the formula websites. As the following passage makes clear, the current scientific view suggests that prebiotics are one component among many others and that these components interact with the infant's developing immune system in complicated ways that are not yet fully understood. Specifically, as described in Lawrence and Pane's literature review:

Within breast milk there are a number of factors that one could consider as acting as part of the infant's innate immune system. This was reviewed at a symposium on "Innate Immunity and Human Milk" as part of the Experimental Biology meeting in April, 2004. Newburg referred to intrinsic components of milk or partially digested products of human milk, which have local antipathogenic effects that supplement the infant's innate immunity. This includes substances that function as prebiotics (substances that enhance the growth of probiotics or beneficial microflora), free fatty acids (FFA), monoglycerides, antimicrobial peptides, and human milk glycans, which bind diarrheal pathogens. In addition to these, there are other factors within breast milk that support or act in concert with the infant's innate immune system including bifidus factor, lysozyme, lactoperoxidase, lactoferrin, lipoprotein lipase, and even epidermal growth factor, which may stimulate the maturation of the gastrointestinal epithelium as a barrier. Newburg also proposed that some factors in milk, which may have no demonstrated immunologic effect when tested alone, may have measurable effects in vivo after digestion or in combination with other factors in breast milk or in the intestine.[28]

Although it might be tempting to view the current discourse on both sides as a straightforward example of the ways in which stakeholders on all sides of a scientific controversy can, in Fahnestock's words, "accommodate" the facts to get their desired message across to specific audiences, I would argue there is something more going on here.[29] There are important differences in the manner in which each side provides scientific information to its target audience, not just in the content provided or in how the evidence is interpreted. That "something more" is what I refer to as viral rhetoric: just as a virus cannot reproduce without inhabiting a host cell, the particular form of rhetoric that formula companies are using to tout the immune-protective qualities of their products could not be persuasive without replicating key ideas from its host rhetoric. The claims that formula companies are currently making about their new enhancements could not be rhetorically successful if the scientific understanding of breast milk's immune-protective properties had not advanced to its current state of sophistication and if today's general public was not widely informed about this scientific knowledge. Because human milk's immune-protective qualities have received so much scientific attention in recent years, formula companies are able to identify specific elements of human milk that are understood to provide some form of immune protection, add these to their products, and then claim that infant formula is closer to human milk than ever before.

Contrasting Rhetorical Frameworks

How are formula companies able to get away with these rhetorical moves? Why can formula companies' websites make all of these claims about the health benefits of the products they sell without citing any scientific research to back up the claims? And why do pro-breastfeeding messages, even when intended for nonexpert audiences, often provide citations to scientific articles to back up their claims? Keeping in mind that rhetorical situation is not a static container or a fixed arena in which rhetorical activity takes place, we might say a closer look reveals more than one situation at issue here—to adopt Edbauer's term *ecology*, the rhetorics of breastfeeding and formula operate in very different ecologies, even if they often seem to present to the public a static situation of choice between relative equals. We cannot just say that arguments on each side invoke different kinds of evidence or that they view the evidence differently and then translate it to various audiences in a linear manner. Rather, arguments on each side relate to the scientific knowledge in a different way, with pro-breastfeeding arguments being in a position that requires them to cite the evidence more directly and transparently. Even though these arguments sometimes take on nonscientific forms that have emotional appeals, like the NBAC campaign images, the relevant scientific evidence can always be tracked down, and careful readers can evaluate that evidence for themselves.

In current formula rhetoric, by contrast, Edbauer's metaphor of viral rhetoric is more appropriate.[30] Discourse such as that found on the formula websites mimics the scientific pro-breastfeeding rhetoric, picking up on bits and pieces of that rhetoric and emphasizing the components of human milk that formula manufacturers have supposedly been successful at replicating. Then they portray the infant's immune system as if those components are the most important part, even though current scientific evidence does not necessarily support that notion. In other words, the discourse on both sides has continued to evolve, and, most notably, just like some viruses can mutate to adapt to new circumstances, formula companies have found ways to adapt their discourse so it can compete (at least for general audiences) with the findings about human milk's unique immune-protective qualities—findings that have led to greater conviction among experts in recent years and thus to more powerful arguments in favor of breastfeeding.

Even though each type of discourse seems neutrally to convey or translate a preexisting set of scientific facts, this neutrality is an illusion. As these "facts" are communicated, they are offered in the context of a complex rhetorical ecology that shapes them but is at the same time continually created and recreated by the circulation of these facts. And in that rhetorical situation, or ecology, the seemingly stable entities of human milk and formula are continually constructed and reconstructed in different ways because the two discourses play by different rules. This contrast can be illustrated in more depth by looking at two recent instances in which advocates of breastfeeding and bottle-feeding have been called on to defend the claims they are making.

Perhaps the most visible controversy surrounding breastfeeding promotion in recent years has been that which surrounded the NBAC. As we have seen above, after extensive focus-group research with groups of mothers who represented various demographics in the United States, the National Ad Council commissioned design of a series of ads that were intended to communicate the message that formula-feeding is dangerous to infants. Just before the ads were scheduled to be released for public viewing, formula companies lobbied the Department of Health and Human Services and succeeded at forcing the campaign developers to tone down the ads. As noted above, the issue on which the controversy hinged was once again accusations that the scientific evidence in support of claims about breastfeeding's health benefits was not convincing enough. Specifically, in a letter to Tommy Thompson dated February 17, 2004, a representative of the formula industry named Clayton Yeutter expressed the industry's disapproval of the pro-breastfeeding ads. Yeutter took issue with the "risk based" focus of the campaign, but his argument ultimately rested on a questioning of the science on which the ads were based: "The infant formula industry and others question the scientific validity of these claims, and they certainly generate skepticism from me as a father and grandfather."[31]

Because formula has long been classified as a food product instead of a drug, formula companies are subject to much less stringent regulations on what they can say and are therefore not obligated to provide any scientific support for the claims that they make, even when those claims appear to translate the most recent scientific evidence into terms that nonexperts can easily understand. As is stated on the FDA website, "because infant formula is a food, the laws and regulations governing foods apply to infant formula."[32] When we look more closely at the site's discussion of regulations, we see the agency's focus is on quality assurance, food safety, avoiding contamination, and so on—all important concerns, of course, but very different from the concerns pertinent to the FDA's regulation of drugs. Specifically, for infant formula there is no mention of efficacy, no requirement for clinically randomized trials that would demonstrate whether these immune-system boosters actually work to reduce infections and to increase health in real populations of babies. Yet we continually make demands for increasingly certain evidence when scientific claims are made about human milk's health benefits. So when Similac's advertising materials claim that its EarlyShield additives support immune-system growth and functioning, there is no requirement to support this claim with any scientific evidence.

Further complicating the issue of infant formula with regard to FDA regulation, some of the recent additives to formula, such as prebiotics that are claimed to support immune-system growth and functioning, are regulated as nutritional supplements, even though formula itself is considered a food. However, it is important to note that there is still no requirement to provide scientific evidence for the kind of claims that Similac is making, for instance, about the immune protection afforded by a product such as EarlyShield. With regard to this matter, the FDA website simply says that "manufacturers must make sure that product label information is truthful and not misleading."[33] As further explained at the FDA website, supplements have been regulated separately from foods since 1994. The following text at the FDA site explains this 1994 law: "In October 1994, the Dietary Supplement Health and Education Act (DSHEA) was signed into law by President Clinton. Before this time, dietary supplements were subject to the same regulatory requirements as were other foods. This new law, which amended the Federal Food, Drug, and Cosmetic Act, created a new regulatory framework for the safety and labeling of dietary supplements."

Under DSHEA, a firm is responsible for determining that the dietary supplements it manufactures or distributes are safe and that any representations or claims made about them are substantiated by adequate evidence to show that they are not false or misleading. This means that dietary supplements do not need approval from the FDA before they are marketed. Except in the case of a new dietary ingredient, where pre-market review for safety data and other information is required by law, a firm does not have to provide the FDA with the evidence it relies on to substantiate safety or effectiveness before or after it markets its products.

Also, manufacturers do not need to register themselves nor their dietary supplement products with the FDA before producing or selling them. Currently, there are no FDA regulations specific to dietary supplements that establish a minimum standard of practice for manufacturing dietary supplements. However, the FDA intends to issue regulations on good manufacturing practices that will focus on practices to ensure the identity, purity, quality, strength, and composition of dietary supplements. At present, the manufacturer is responsible for establishing its own manufacturing-practice guidelines to ensure that the dietary supplements it produces are safe and contain the ingredients listed on the label.[34]

This legal language is important because it stipulates that the formula manufacturers themselves are responsible for ensuring the safety of any new ingredients they add to their products and that they are not obligated to make their evidence available for scrutiny from the FDA or any other regulating body. It is also important because it completely sidesteps the issue of efficacy. Although formula companies are supposed to provide labels that are "truthful and not misleading," they have a lot of leeway to determine for themselves what would constitute truthful versus misleading information.

Thus, a few years ago, when formula companies wanted to add prebiotics to their formulas, all they had to do was conduct research to prove the new additives were safe and then report the results of such research to the FDA in something called a "Generally Recognized as Safe" (GRAS) determination. In the case of prebiotics, this additive was the subject of a GRAS determination in 2007. The new component was described as follows in the FDA document: "The subject of the GRAS determination, galacto-oligosaccharide (GOS), is a nondigestible carbohydrate that selectively stimulates the growth and/or activity of one or a limited number of bacteria in the colon. The intended effect of GOS is to provide a dietary source of this oligosaccharide."[35]

This document submitted to the FDA provided a far more in-depth explanation of the scientific reasoning supporting the formula companies' claims about its new additive's immune-protective qualities than a reader will ever find at Similac's or Enfamil's website. Based on the FDA document, we can surmise that the "prebiotics" added to the newest brands of formula are meant to replicate the immune-protective qualities of similar elements that have long been known to exist in human milk. However, it is important to note that the entire FDA document is aimed at proving the safety of the ingredient, and thus, it reports a great deal of evidence in support of its claim that this ingredient will not harm an infant who digests it. Although there is some discussion of the reasons why the ingredient is postulated to offer benefits, there is no evidence to demonstrate that it does in fact offer these benefits—no randomized clinical trials, as would be required for approval of a new pharmaceutical product, and none of the large-scale studies that are routinely demanded to support claims about breastfeeding's health benefits. The document cites studies on rats and mice to prove that the prebiotics lead to greater concentrations of the so-called healthy bacteria in the rodents' stools. But, as we have seen, we have long known these bacteria exist in breastfed infants as well, yet that knowledge has never been enough—there are always further demands for additional research to prove definitively the related health benefits in live populations, and these demands take on different forms as the conversation among scientific experts continues to develop.

This contrast between the manner in which scientific evidence was provided, questioned, and evaluated in two recent instances involving human milk and infant formula illustrates how the discussion of breast versus bottle-feeding has been framed from its beginning, suggesting a perspective on this set of issues that has not yet been addressed in current feminist critiques of breastfeeding discourse. The review article cited in the AAP poster offers further insight into how the battle lines have been drawn in this discussion, with breastfeeding advocates in the defensive position. Specifically, the authors described the review's purpose as follows:

> The intention of this review was to discuss important concepts related to the role breastfeeding plays in the normal development of the infant's immune system and the protection afforded the infant against infectious diseases during infancy and childhood, while the infant's immune system is still maturing. The discussion should provide ample evidence to support the current recommendations for 6 months of exclusive breastfeeding for all infants, help all health care providers adequately inform families of the real immune benefits of breastfeeding, and strongly support and advocate for breastfeeding in their day-to-day care of children.[36]

This language further suggests how advocates of breastfeeding have felt the need, once again, to compile and present all the available evidence. Even despite the rhetorical success that might be indicated by the 1997 and 2005 AAP policy statements, conversations about the health benefits and risks of breast- and bottle-feeding continue to evolve, and many of the same historical tendencies we have discussed still persist.

Historical Perspectives

It is interesting that the emergence of this viral rhetoric seems to be rather recent. If we look back at rhetorical strategies that formula companies were using just a few years ago, before breastfeeding promotion became as bold and widespread as it is today, we see something quite different. In this relatively brief period, we see a rather dramatic shift from a line of reasoning best summarized as "breast is best, but if you have to use formula, choose ours" (common during the 1990s) to "our product might be just as good as human milk because we've added such and such." Looking at Similac's previous websites, which can be accessed through WaybackMachine,[37] it appears that the immune-supporting additives first started to be promoted in 2005,[38] and that was the same time that the depiction of formula's relationship to human milk also changed. It was also at about the same time that the NBAC ads started circulating and that what I have called the topos of breastfeeding as the norm started to evolve into the topos of formula as risky. It is interesting that formula companies' advertising expenditures also increased drastically around this time.[39] As for Enfamil, the shift seemed to have occurred slightly later. This company seems to have just begun advertising their Triple Health Guard formula in 2009, and we see a similar rhetorical shift in their depiction of breast versus bottle at that same time as well.[40]

If we once again take a historical view, it is clear that both companies' citation practices have also undergone some changes in recent years, coinciding with the shift in rhetorical strategies discussed above. In all of the Similac sites dated prior to 2005 (1998–2004), scientific studies were cited to support the claims that the company was making about its additives at that time, which included DHA and another product that they claimed would improve the infant's bone density. But in 2005, when the company started promoting EarlyShield, the scientific references went away. As for Enfamil, their older sites were divided into sections for parents and health-care professionals. The health-care-professional portions of the sites provided references to scientific studies, but the parent portions did not.[41] Furthermore, sometime within the last five years, there has been a general shift in both companies' advertising messages from "breast milk is best, but if you don't want to or can't breast-feed, then ask your doctor about formula" to "our product is getting closer to human milk." For the Similac site, this shift might be concurrent with the new immune-system additives and also concurrent with the decision to stop providing scientific references; for Enfamil, it is harder to trace exactly when this rhetorical shift occurred.

In light of these recent changes in formula-promotion tactics, the current similarities in public discourse on breast- and bottle-feeding might suggest that the terms of the debate have shifted to favor breastfeeding. Whereas formula companies used to be able to promote their product as an acceptable substitute when breastfeeding fails, this strategy started to lose its effectiveness when, a few years ago, breastfeeding started to be promoted more aggressively with reference to specific immune-system benefits supported by increasingly solid scientific evidence. As a result, we might argue, formula companies have had to find ways to make their own arguments sound more scientific, and they have had to find an answer to the continually increasing evidence of human milk's immune-protective properties.

As we have seen above, in the time period since commercially produced formulas have become widely available the rhetorical situation "breast or bottle" has taken on a shape that has led scientific and medical experts who advocate breastfeeding to be on the defensive. We saw also that, as a result of these expert advocates' efforts, breastfeeding seems to have made great strides in this ongoing contest, especially in recent years, and formula companies' current rhetorical efforts might be seen as a necessary response to that advancement. A survey designed to track the effectiveness of the NBAC ads found that the percentage of U.S. adults who either knew that current medical recommendations encourage mothers to breastfeed exclusively for the first six months or indicated that the recommended duration is longer than six months increased from 52 percent in 2004 to 63 percent in 2005.[42] Some of the recent statistics also suggest that breastfeeding rates are on the rise, at least in the earliest phases of newborns' lives, if not in later months. These various occurrences would seem to demand that formula companies change their tactics, and, in fact, this has been suggested by a recent California WIC Association study that made the following accusations: "As the U.S. birth rate levels off, growth in the domestic infant formula market is primarily being driven by price increases, not by the quantity of formula sold." To maintain profitability, formula manufacturers have raised their prices by creating a dizzying array of new product lines and additives that come with attractive—though scientifically questionable—health claims.[43]

According to these perspectives, we might conclude that the whole rhetorical situation has been powerfully shaped by scientific understandings of human milk's role in the immune system that have taken hold since the 1970s. On both sides the stakes have risen, with great pressure to sound scientific. On the breastfeeding side we see a shift toward emphasizing the risks of formula use rather than just benefits of breastfeeding. On the formula side we see a shift from "breastfeeding is best but if you have to bottle-feed, then choose our product" to "our product might be just as good as human milk." Given the extent to which infant feeding has become medicalized in the United States since the mid–twentieth century, it is not surprising to see discourse on both breastfeeding and formula connecting claims more solidly to scientific evidence than they have done in the past.[44]

In rhetorical terms, as the topos of breastfeeding as the norm evolves into the topos of formula as risky, discourses on both sides appear to be forging stronger rhetorical connections to science. This shift could be occurring because the amount of scientific evidence that appears to prove breastfeeding's health benefits has continued to increase in recent years, which has caused the stakes to rise in the ongoing scientific discussion that frames mothers' apparent choices between breast and bottle. In the case of discourses that promote breastfeeding, the pressure to cite definitive scientific evidence has continued to increase, continuing the historical trajectory charted above. Furthermore, as the topos of formula as risky has taken form, there has also been a shift toward emphasizing the risks of formula rather than just the benefits of human milk. In the case of discourses that promote infant formula, important tactical changes have occurred as well: formula companies have developed new products that they are now claiming provide immune-protective qualities similar to those in human milk. This development has led to fundamental shifts in their overall marketing strategies.

Mothers' Perspectives

Listening to the comments of mothers who participated in the nine focus groups conducted from July to December 2008 provides additional insights into the manner in which formula discourse is functioning as a viral rhetoric.[45] Our interdisciplinary team used the following eleven questions to spark discussion about participants' perceptions of information they had received about infant feeding:

- What do you think are the most important differences between breast- and bottle-feeding?
- Can you recall where you got these impressions about breast- and bottle-feeding? Are they based on your own experiences? Experiences of friends and relatives? The media? Health professionals?
- How many people do you know who have breastfed their babies? Bottle-fed?
- What do you think it means when someone talks about having a "good baby"? Does feeding have anything to do with this?
- At what age should a baby be weaned from the breast? From the bottle? What's the best time to start solid foods, and why?
- Where do you usually turn for information on health or medical topics? What kinds of information, if any, have these sources offered you on infant feeding?
- When do you think most women make decisions about infant feeding (early in pregnancy, late in pregnancy, after birth, etc.)?
- What do you think are the reasons why women decide to breastfeed or bottle-feed?
- Do you think it's possible to go back to work and still continue breastfeeding?
- Do you think your own mother heard different advice about infant feeding from what you are hearing today? If so, why?

- What do you think about breastfeeding in public?

Only two of the questions in this list pertain specifically to breastfeeding: question 9, which asks about continuing to breastfeed while working outside the home, and question 11, which asks about breastfeeding in public. All of the other questions ask mothers to comment on infant feeding in general and include specific prompts to this effect. However, without exception, the conversations in these groups naturally developed toward a focus on information about breastfeeding rather than bottle-feeding.

Whereas these mothers frequently mentioned that the "breast is best" message appears to be everywhere, they rarely made any specific mention of the nature or quality of information that is communicated to mothers about formula-feeding. The following are some sample quotations from the focus-group participants to illustrate this point:

> "I got my subscription to *Baby Talk* magazine and *American Baby.* And both of those—breast, breast, breast, breast, breast. Now, they talk about formula, but I read. I read everything, every word, cover to cover. And it's breasts. You know, they say, 'Well, if you must formula feed,' . . . and then *Parents* magazine that I'm getting now is pretty much the same way. And women are coming to places like this and they're getting those magazines (and they're free); free is always easier to get a hold of. And that's pushing. So I think that's having a lot of influence on them." (Jill)

> "Everywhere you look, especially if you're in our programs in the community, . . . any hospital is going to tell you to breastfeed. WIC, if you're on WIC, they're going to push breastfeeding. So you hear it from everywhere. . . . There are signs everywhere. I almost think you could put them by the stop sign and they would be just as effective [laughter]. You walk into the WIC office and there's this chick with her boob out and the baby's on it. . . . I was just in there today and that's what it is. Even now, I'm just two months and they're [asking] are you going to breastfeed or bottle-feed? I don't know. I can't think that far. I'm still having to recuperate from the shock. My second one is just five months. . . . So, yeah, I mean, they might as well just stick [the signs] on the bathroom stalls. I mean, that's how it is. Anywhere you go. Especially if you get any help from anywhere." (Tracy)

> "It seems like [the "breast is best" message] is everywhere. Everybody has an opinion. Like, even public service announcements on TV. And books. At the OBGYN, while you're sitting there, the poster." (Nancy)

> "So I guess, if even the formula companies say that—that breast milk is best—I guess that's just fact now, I guess." (Angelica)

As suggested by these quotations, participants in these focus groups almost unanimously agreed that the "breast is best" message is highly visible today.

Furthermore, in every group there were several participants who could name specific health benefits that they had learned breastfeeding offers to the mother or infant. In addition to frequent mention of the prevalence of the "breast is best" message, the group conversations often turned to other aspects of breastfeeding information; in many cases participants became quite passionate and the discussion quite vibrant. Participants sometimes complained that today's infant-feeding information is "biased" toward breastfeeding or that those who communicate infant-feeding information have an "agenda" that favors breastfeeding. They sometimes also complained about the imbalance of all the messages everywhere urging them to breastfeed and the lack of information available to help them address breastfeeding problems after the baby was born.

A few mothers mentioned receiving free formula samples in the mail or at the hospital, but, for the most part, when formula-feeding was mentioned in these focus groups, it was depicted as relatively uninteresting or unproblematic: the foolproof option that does not require any specialized information for success. Whereas participants told countless stories about situations (either their own or of someone they knew) in which breastfeeding "didn't work out," they were almost unanimous in expressing the idea that bottle-feeding was a dependable fallback and that, in contrast to breastfeeding, even mothers who had never done it before would be able to do it without any specialized information or additional support.

As Jill, a focus-group participant, said, "it's easy to make the bottle, you just pop the top." Others echoed this impression of bottle-feeding with comments such as the following:

> "Here I am rocking, praying, and crying-sobbing because my baby was so hungry. There's a can of formula sitting right there. I popped that bottle in his mouth and he was happy, slept through the night. I was scared because he was so happy." (Tracy)

> "The same way that it was taken away from you, you weren't able to breastfeed. I couldn't . . . breastfeed her. She wouldn't latch on. She wouldn't, she just decided that it wasn't for her. It was her decision, so you know. And formula is more expensive, but like you said, it's just easier." (Danielle)

> "Well, yeah, I've been reading a lot of books just to pass the time, and learn a lot of different things that other moms have experienced. . . . But my family, personally, tells me that it always hurts too much so they always go back to formula after about three months. But after hearing all the benefits of breastfeeding, I'm definitely going to do it." (Theresa)

> "I think most mothers probably say, 'Oh, I want to nurse!' You know, but it's not as easy. I know for myself and some friends, especially with

their first child when you don't really know what you're doing, it's really hard. And it's just easier to stop at that point and pick up a bottle." (Angelica)

The stark contrast between mothers' perceptions of information on breast- and bottle-feeding, as well as the impression that breastfeeding information is far more prevalent than bottle-feeding information, is interesting for a couple of reasons. First, there is a contradiction between perceptions of the problems that arise from breastfeeding and those that arise from formula-feeding. The problems affiliated with breastfeeding—everything from inconvenience to fussy babies to sore nipples and "not enough milk"—seemed to suggest automatically the need to switch to formula. By contrast, when mothers in these groups spoke of problems that, according to current expert discourses, are caused or exacerbated by formula use—diaper rash, allergies, constipation, and the like—the blame was never placed on formula per se. Rather, mothers were more likely to speak of the need to switch to a different brand of formula or just to accept that these conditions were a normal part of babyhood. This contradictory perception is interesting because it indicates how far our society is from treating breastfeeding as the normal feeding method, even though this is the official stance of the medical community now.

Second, and more germane to our focus on viral rhetoric, these contradictory perceptions of breastfeeding and bottle-feeding information do not correspond with what we know about dollars spent on formula advertising versus breastfeeding promotion in the United States each year. Some of the most recent available estimates suggest that formula companies spent at least forty-six million dollars on television, print, and radio advertisements in 2004, which is a dramatic increase from the thirty million dollars estimated for 2000. Furthermore, from 1999 to 2004, the number of television and print ads for infant formula reportedly increased from seven thousand to ten thousand, and more than forty thousand television and print ads for infant formula appeared during this period.[46] Total advertising expenditures for the formula industry, including all the free samples and promotional materials sent to physicians, clinics, and hospitals, have been estimated at two to three billion dollars per year.[47] These increased advertising expenditures on the part of formula companies are largely understood as a response to stepped-up efforts at breastfeeding promotion. Although breastfeeding advocacy organizations typically do not have as much money to spend on advertising, some of the recent campaigns have been quite expensive. For instance, the recent "Born to Breastfeed" campaign reportedly cost about forty million dollars.[48]

Thus, both parties in the ongoing "contest" between breast and bottle have increased their spending in recent years, and both are spending a lot of money, but breastfeeding organizations are certainly not spending more than formula companies. Nonetheless, it is noteworthy that not one participant in our focus groups ever said that she was constantly urged to buy formula. Not a single participant said that formula companies who mailed free samples to her home had an "agenda." By contrast, participants routinely made remarks such as these with regard to breastfeeding information.

The fact that many of the pro-formula claims are functioning as a viral rhetoric that mimics key elements from pro-breastfeeding discourse might explain why mothers who participated in these focus groups feel this message is so pervasive; they are likely hearing about human milk's immune-protective benefits from both sides in the debate. The surface similarities between current breastfeeding and bottle-feeding discourse mask some fundamental differences that could easily be overlooked by the typical consumer of both kinds of information. Most important, one thing that has remained constant from the historical situation we reviewed earlier is that the two sides in this controversy still play by different rules, so the formula discourse does not have to provide scientific evidence to support its claims, whereas breastfeeding advocates are required to provide documentation—a difference that is likely to go unnoticed by some consumers of this information. Despite the impression that the "breast is best" message is everywhere, then, and despite the fact that the general status and visibility of breastfeeding's health benefits in the United States seem to have increased in recent years, there are still important fundamental differences between the rhetorical tactics used on both sides, and these differences relate in interesting ways to the recent history of U.S. infant-feeding controversies.

Viral Rhetorics in the Kairology of Infant Feeding

Although the promotional texts we have compared provide a useful starting place for understanding the breast–bottle debate, it is important to look at such texts not in isolation but as existing within a rhetorical ecology not entirely of their own making. In addition to the fact that they exist within these ecologies, these texts produce these rhetorical ecologies, or perpetuate them, through discursive actions in themselves. Furthermore, the two kinds of discourses are caught up in very different rhetorical ecologies. As we have seen repeatedly, those who advocate breastfeeding have continually had to fight against negative perceptions, which have assumed various different forms over the decades. Thus, advocates of breastfeeding are forced to provide more and more evidence for their claims that human milk is fundamentally different from formula and contains properties that offer unique health benefits. Formula companies have only had to prove that their products will not harm infants, so the bar is much lower. This is now especially true because recent legislation allows all of the new additives to formula to be classified as supplements, and, since 1994, supplements are subject to less stringent regulations than drugs.

In sum, then, even though discourse on both sides of the breast–bottle debate might seem to convey scientific facts neutrally, the authors of such discourses are actually playing by dramatically different rules. It is not just a situation of scientific uncertainty, in which the evidence is conflicting and each side selects the evidence that best supports its cause (which is a commonsense way of thinking about scientific controversies such as environmentalism). Rather, the playing field is unevenly constructed so that arguments on each side are required to provide fundamentally different kinds of evidence for their claims. If breastfeeding discourse is much more transparent, that is because proponents of breastfeeding have been forced to make their evidence available for public scrutiny, and, because it is available for public scrutiny, it is continually questioned, and breastfeeding advocates are forced to provide stronger evidence. They have been required to provide more stringent evidence at every step of the way. If breastfeeding discourse today sometimes seems overly strident, or seems as if it has an agenda, that is because anyone who has advocated breastfeeding in recent decades has had to do so from a defensive position, and they have had a lot of momentum to fight against from the other side. If many mothers today feel like the "breast is best" message is saturating the airwaves, it is probably, at least in part, due to the rhetorical phenomena we have exposed.

As we have seen, despite the progress that we seem to have made in regard to our understanding and appreciation of human milk, the contest is far from over. The current rhetorical situation of infant feeding is powerfully shaped by scientific understandings of human milk's role in the immune system that have taken hold since the 1970s. We have noted also the rhetorical significance of these new scientific understandings—the extent to which they have altered the framework in which arguments about infant feeding are produced and the rules that such arguments have to follow. This, however, does not mean the debate is over or the controversy settled. Rather, the scientific understandings are in themselves moving targets, continually in flux and always changing. They constitute a powerful force at the moment—a force that has become increasingly prevalent since the 1970s. But if we look at the whole situation in terms of rhetorical ecology, as defined by Edbauer, we can see those scientific understandings as one powerful element among many others. Even though arguments on both sides in the debate are shaped by this force, the shaping unfolds in very different ways.

Although the general contours of the infant-feeding situation have continued to be defined by a breast—bottle choice, as we have looked more closely, we have seen some subtle changes occurring in the exact manner in which that choice is framed. Some fundamental elements of the larger situation have stayed the same, but the increased amount and quality of scientific knowledge about human milk's immune-protective qualities and the changes in medical policy have altered this larger rhetorical situation in some subtle yet important ways, causing discourse on both sides to undergo some fundamental changes.

The findings of our rhetorical analysis are noteworthy for several reasons. First, they might provide a partial explanation for the impression that "breast is best" is everywhere and the widespread knowledge of specific health benefits that breast milk offers. Ironically, one might even argue that formula-advertising dollars are actually helping spread the "breast is best" message through what I have called a viral rhetoric that disseminates specific information about the ways in which human milk is understood to enhance the infant's immune system. Second, the findings shed new light on the current feminist conversations and disagreements regarding the science behind breastfeeding. These fundamental differences between the ways in which arguments are made about human milk and about formula have not received much attention from feminist scholars. Feminist scholars have focused mostly on the perceived bias in breastfeeding discourse or they have treated the scientific and expert discourses as a black box, without much critical attention at all. But the disparity that became evident in our historical analysis persists in today's discourse, even though it is taking on different forms. To echo the findings set forth above, when we look behind this apparently smooth connection between medical recommendations and scientific evidence, we see some interesting differences in the science–medicine relationship as it exists in the case of breastfeeding discourse and formula discourse. In actuality, breastfeeding and formula discourse are fundamentally different—far more so than is suggested by the tendency to portray them as relative equals, each with their own pros and cons, or by formula companies' current attempts to portray formula as increasingly similar to human milk. Although discourse on both forms of infant feeding might seem neutrally to translate recent scientific findings into terms that nonexperts can understand and apply in their own lives, we have seen that they are two very different types of discourse that relate to their nonexpert audiences in fundamentally different ways in a rhetorical situation still in flux and subject to change. We turn now to take a more expansive view of the current rhetorical situation by considering forms of infant-feeding information that mothers are receiving from less official sources.

5

....

Rhetorical Agency and Resistance
in the Context of Infant Feeding

> You're challenging the person who's taking care of your baby. . . .
> It's almost like when I told the dental hygienist that I wanted her
> to change her gloves. . . . The thought that she had a sharp instru-
> ment went through my head. . . . Do I really want to say this?
>
> "KATHERINE," in an interview, May 8, 2000

As we continue to analyze how the breast–bottle controversy impacts the
mothers targeted by today's messages about infant feeding, we turn to consider the messages that women are hearing about infant feeding from friends,
relatives, and health-care professionals, and through other informal means of
communication. These diverse messages can be usefully understood as what
J. Blake Scott calls "disciplinary rhetorics"—that is, as "discursive bodies of
persuasion that work with extrarhetorical actors to shape subjects and to work
on and through bodies."[1] The concept of disciplinary rhetoric derives from
Michel Foucault's concept of disciplinary power, a uniquely modern form of
power that emerged in Western civilization during the eighteenth century as
part of an array of political, institutional, and cultural shifts occurring at that
time. Although disciplinary power, as Foucault describes it, is invisible, in contrast to the more obvious forms of power that preceded it (corporal punish-
ment, for instance), its ultimate effect on those individuals who are subject to
it (e.g., people who seek medical advice on a topic such as infant feeding) can

be a heightened visibility in relation to institutions such as medicine. That is, although institutions today do not generally threaten individuals with physical reprimands, they do closely scrutinize our behavior, and this close scrutiny constitutes a form of power that, Foucault would say, we need to take seriously in its own right.

As Foucault explains in *Discipline and Punish,* "in discipline, it is the subjects who have to be seen. Their visibility assures the hold of the power that is exercised over them. It is the fact of being constantly seen, of being able always to be seen, that maintains the disciplined individual in his subjection."[2] Thus, in Foucault's explanation, disciplinary power not only acts on individuals but actually makes us who we are by training us to monitor ourselves according to the truths that disciplinary institutions such as the medical profession establish. This means that normalizing claims about an aspect of life such as infant feeding never exist strictly in the realm of scientific or medical truth but are always brought to bear on the bodies of subjects in a manner that blurs the boundaries traditionally believed to exist among the realms of science, politics, and the economy.

Communication researchers have used Foucault's concept of disciplinary power to understand the complex dynamics and power relations that can arise when technical information on a wide array of subjects is communicated from experts to nonexperts. Communication scholars have, for example, used Foucault's concepts to analyze the medical and legal rhetorics of HIV testing, infertility treatment and insurance coverage, and home birth and midwifery.[3] Although the subject matter of such analyses is diverse, the important idea that emerges from them is that when technical information on subjects such as these is communicated to the nonexperts, such as patients and consumers who use it to make decisions about treatments or other serious matters, this is not a neutral communicative act but rather a rhetorical situation that is infused with power. Along these lines, Foucault urges us to acknowledge that "power and knowledge directly imply one another; that there is no power relation without the correlative constitution of a field of knowledge, nor any knowledge that does not presuppose and constitute at the same time power relations."[4]

One of the most important questions that continue to emerge from such analyses, and a question that directly relates to the experiences of breastfeeding women, is that of individual agency. Although disciplinary rhetorics are acknowledged as intensely powerful in their ability to shape reality, it is also obvious that individuals possess the capacity to take meaningful action from within the grid of meaning that is established through disciplinary power.[5] Although it is clear, for instance, that the physician who communicates expert knowledge to a patient derives a certain form of power over the patient, we also know that the patient can question the physician's advice in a number of ways. The patient's actions might include direct questioning, seeking a second opinion from another physician, or possibly turning to the Internet. Despite this awareness of capacity for rhetorical agency and resistance, however, there remains some uncertainty about the precise nature and limitations of such actions. Although it is well established that subjects are capable of "rhetorical negotiation" or "choices between competing alternatives,"[6] it is also clear that this ability to choose has limits. For instance, a patient might encounter material limitations, such as health insurance that makes it difficult to obtain a second opinion; intellectual limitations, such as the inability to understand the information that is found through Internet searches; or personal limitations, such as feelings of fear and a reluctance to go too far in questioning medical authority. In rhetorical terms, previous communication research has made clear that we should not understand rhetorical agency as simply a two-way struggle between the individual and the ideological force of institutions. Rather, individuals' rhetorical actions are always grounded in the same disciplinary rhetorics that circumscribe an experience such as infant feeding.[7] In other words, individuals might resist certain elements of disciplinary rhetoric, but they never escape the grid of disciplinary power altogether.

Taking these ideas about rhetorical agency, resistance, and disciplinary rhetoric as a starting place, we shall look at some of the ways in which women are grappling with the troubling situations that can emerge from their interactions with today's expert discourses on infant feeding. Our analysis is based on the interviews and focus groups conducted in two different locations over the last several years. Participants include a wide range of mothers who have had an even wider range of experiences with breastfeeding. The initial interviews involved breastfeeding advocates who worked in various capacities to support mothers and assist them when they encountered problems, but since then the pool of research participants has expanded to include mothers without any specialized expertise in infant feeding: some of these mothers have breastfed for various lengths of time, some tried breastfeeding and then switched to the bottle, and others bottle-fed from the beginning. Collectively, the data presented suggest that to follow current official medical guidelines on breastfeeding, guidelines advising that infants should be breastfed for at least one year, women often have to resist various other elements of medical discourse and larger cultural perceptions that directly contradict these official guidelines. Specifically, in many of the examples presented, women received messages from health-care professionals or other sources that incorrectly advised them to wean or to take other actions that interfere with successful lactation. Thus, based on these examples, one can conclude that, with regard to breastfeeding, the power of disciplinary rhetoric resides not in any single message about what women should do but in the mixed messages that circumscribe what their bodies can do. From a feminist perspective, this observation is important because it emphasizes that the embodied experience of breastfeeding in contemporary U.S. culture places women in a troubling position in what Carl G. Herndl and Adele C. Licona call the "network of semiotic, material, and . . . intentional elements and relational practices" that circumscribe this aspect of life.[8]

After establishing this rhetorical dynamic as it exists in relation to breastfeeding, it is useful to expose some of the strategies that research participants have used to take action in the face of the problematic rhetorical context that continues to discourage breastfeeding even though official medical recommendations encourage it. In some cases, women are able to realize their own intentions successfully in the context of disciplinary rhetorics—for example, by seeking alternatives to medical advice they perceive as incorrect or by continuing to breastfeed even when members of their immediate social circles do not approve it. Echoing the findings of previous communication research, these women's individual acts of resistance suggest that systemwide change is possible, although we must expect that change to be difficult and to take a long time. In theoretical terms, our analysis reinforces the idea that individual agency and the ideological force of disciplinary rhetorics are inextricably linked and adds to our understanding by taking a close look at the relationship between the rhetorical agency involved in acts of resistance and the ultimate outcomes of such acts. Specifically, the acts of resistance that interviewees describe begin as active selection among discursive alternatives—the kind of rhetorical negotiation that might be construed as the occupation of preexisting positions within a grid of disciplinary power rather than true resistance. However, when we examine the effects of these women's acts of resistance, we see something more than the occupation of predefined positions in a grid: we see that resistance can, in the words of Barbara Biesecker, "defy translation, throw sense off track, and, thus, short-circuit the system through which sense is made."[9] Examining this rhetorical phenomenon as it relates to infant feeding is important because it emphasizes how unpredictable the outcomes of such actions can be. Even when sense is disrupted, a positive outcome is not guaranteed, and, in fact, such disruption can occasionally lead to social sanctions against the perceived offender—sanctions that can reinforce the previous "system through which sense is made" and thus negate any effects that might have initially seemed to indicate progress toward positive change.

Breastfeeding Discourse as Disciplinary Rhetoric

The AAP's declaration of breastfeeding as the norm, first established in the 1997 policy statement and reinforced in the 2005 revision of that statement, was, in part, an effort to make infant-feeding information more consistent within the medical community and in the culture at large. As recent historical research has revealed, in the early and mid–twentieth century, U.S. hospitals adopted practices such as separating mothers and infants, enforcing rigid feeding schedules, and offering formula at the first sign of breastfeeding dif-ficulty. Because a mother's milk supply can only be established and main-tained through frequent infant sucking, practices such as these can sabotage breastfeeding by reducing the mother's chances of establishing a sufficient milk supply before she even leaves the hospital. Thus, many scholars believe, breast-feeding mothers have long faced a contradiction: although official medical dis-course has long promoted breastfeeding, bottle-feeding has become accepted as the medical and cultural norm.[10]

In response to this historical context, the AAP's 1997 and 2005 policy statements offer specific advice to govern physicians' and mothers' interpreta-tions of the breastfeeding body—advice that is intended to reassure them in the face of infant behavior that might seem worrisome in a culture accustomed to bottle-fed babies. For instance, the statements affirm that it is normal for breastfed babies to eat frequently, advising mothers to allow their babies to eat "whenever they show signs of hunger" rather than try to adhere to a rigid feed-ing schedule.[11] They spell out what health-care practitioners should expect to see in the normal nursing mother–baby pair. Although these policy statements have achieved a high profile in the medical community and in the popular media, my qualitative research during the last decade suggests that women who attempt to breastfeed today still encounter many of the beliefs that have been affiliated with the long-standing topos of breastfeeding as foundation (which entails a view of bottle-feeding as the norm). These beliefs, although incorrect, are often disguised in medical and cultural practice as neutral scientific truth and are manifested in various ways. In fact, the mothers' stories reported in the focus groups suggest that disciplinary power does not reside exclusively in the language of official medical discourse such as the AAP's 1997 statement but also occurs through convergence of various, often conflicting, messages that mothers still receive from the medical establishment, mass media, and the culture at large.

In theoretical terms, the conflicts that interviewees describe manifest Fou-cault's observations about the connection between power and knowledge—his well-known assertion that power and knowledge are so intimately linked that one cannot exist without the other—expressed in French as *pouvoir-savoir*.[12] Although this French term is usually translated into English as power-knowledge, an alternative translation is useful in explaining the breastfeeding difficulties that many mothers experience. Offering an alternative translation, Gayatri Spivak observes that *pouvoir* means "to be able" as well as "power."[13] When *pouvoir* is translated as to be able, "power names not the imposition of a limit that constrains human thought and action but a being-able that is made

possible by a grid of intelligibility."[14] By adopting this slightly different translation, disciplinary power can be understood not only as dictating what subjects
should do but also as producing the very rhetorical situations in which they act
by specifying what their bodies can do.

Reflecting this idea that disciplinary rhetoric can define what subjects' bodies are capable of doing, many of the women interviewed have suggested that
the conflicting messages women receive sometimes quite literally make breastfeeding impossible. For instance, Sharon, who was a board-certified lactation
consultant in a large urban hospital when she was interviewed, said that in the
hospital where she worked, breastfeeding was still frequently "sabotaged."
That is, even though the AAP's 1997 policy statement stipulates that most
mothers can nourish their babies exclusively through breastfeeding for the first
four to six months of life and advises physicians that supplementary foods
should not be given to newborns "unless a medical indication exists," nurses
sometimes offered bottles of formula anyway.[15] In Sharon's words, "there are
lots of ways that [breastfeeding] can be sabotaged. And certainly I don't want
to give you the wrong impression that it's every nurse who's doing this, . . . but
it is a problem."

Despite the critical tone of Sharon's remarks, health-care practitioners who
offer unnecessary supplements do not necessarily act with the intention of disrupting the breastfeeding relationship. More likely, they offer bottles because
it is convenient and because it accords with past practices. One might say
it is part of health-care professionals' habitus, a repertoire of practices that
have come to seem natural and correct through years of formal training and
repeated observations of their colleagues' accepted ways of doing things.[16]
But regardless of the motivations for it, the breastfeeding advocates interviewed see early supplementation, especially if it occurs without the mother's
knowing about it, as particularly insidious because the breastfeeding relationship is especially vulnerable to disruption in the first few days of an infant's
life.

Offering another example, Jackie, a Leche League leader in a rural Mid-
western area, observed that even within the medical establishment women are
likely to receive advice that contradicts the 1997 statement's guidelines:

> "In the hospitals and in the doctor's office, they're saying the right thing,
> but they don't believe it. And when a mother has a deviation from some-
> thing, it becomes too easy to fall back into their old thing. If the baby's
> glucose is a little off at birth, well, we better give the baby formula. Or
> if the baby's a little jaundiced, rather than looking at all the reasons that
> the baby could be jaundiced that are benign, we immediately suspect it's
> breast milk and tell the mother she can't nurse for twenty-four hours to see
> if that helps."

Jackie went on to indicate that the medical profession is starting to change in this regard, but not as quickly as she would like: "I think the medical profession used to say it's fine if you want to breastfeed. They'd throw a lot of obstacles in your way. They felt the need to quantify everything and measure everything, and expect babies to be on the same schedule as the artificially fed babies were. Since that time, with my own children, I've watched a lot of the rules of how to breastfeed fall by the wayside. . . . And, by the time I had my last one, and currently, it's more, nurse the baby as long as the baby wants to nurse, encourage more frequent feedings if you can. But what's being done that's so frustrating is, it's still just lip service."

Interviewees also frequently mentioned that there is a great deal of variation among hospitals and clinics. As Ellen, also a La Leche League leader, reported, women are likely to get different information depending on whom they ask, because "there's a wide variety of information and in the ways that different facilities deal with it."

More recent interviews have included mothers with a wider range of infant-feeding experiences and who do not possess the same specialized expertise as Sharon, Jackie, or Ellen. The stories of these diverse mothers, many of whom have been hospital patients in the kinds of situations that breastfeeding supporters such as Sharon, Jackie, and Ellen describe, reinforce the observations of lactation consultants and La Leche League leaders and offer another perspective on the function of disciplinary rhetoric. When we hear some of these mothers' experiences, it becomes clear that health-care professionals still have a lot to learn about how to treat the breastfeeding patient. Some of the stories these women have told suggest that, even if health-care professionals are aware of currently accepted facts about the health benefits of breastfeeding, they are not yet accustomed to factoring the breastfeeding relationship into the equation when mothers face different options for treating a given medical condition.

One frequent occurrence, for instance, is that health-care professionals incorrectly advise mothers that they need to wean because a particular medication they have been prescribed will harm the baby. For instance, Carrie was a mother who gave birth in a Lubbock, Texas, hospital in 2001. She described a situation in which she was advised that she had to stop breastfeeding her two-day-old baby for at least twenty-four hours because she had taken a dose of the pain medication Vicodin: "So they wanted to make sure that all the medicine was out of my system before I tried to breastfeed again. So I pumped and threw away the milk. . . . And then I couldn't get her to latch back on. . . . She never latched on after she quit."

Vicodin (the brand name for a narcotic pain medication consisting of hydrocodone and acetominophen) is currently classified as L3, which means "moderately safe," in Thomas Hale's medical reference *Medications and*

Mothers' Milk.[17] Similarly, Lactmed, which is a publicly available online database of information on drug safety for lactating mothers, also characterizes Vicodin as most likely safe, although it recommends a maximum daily dose of 30 mg and advises that the nursing infant should be monitored for "drowsiness, adequate weight gain, and developmental milestones."[18]

Furthermore, recent AAP policy advises that most prescription medications are safe for nursing mothers. For instance, the AAP's 2005 policy statement stipulates that "Although breastfeeding is optimal for infants, there are a few conditions under which breastfeeding may not be in the best interest of the infant."[19] The statement then lists these few contraindications, which include some medical conditions as well as a small number of drugs: "mothers who are receiving diagnostic or therapeutic radioactive isotopes or have had exposure to radioactive materials (for as long as there is radioactive material in the milk); mothers who are receiving antimetabolites or chemotherapeutic agents or a small number of other medications until they clear the milk; mothers who are using drugs of abuse ('street drugs')."[20] Vicodin is not mentioned in this AAP statement as a contraindication to breastfeeding.

The AAP Committee on Drugs also has a policy statement, last updated in 2001, that offers practical guidelines such as advising physicians to question whether a particular drug is absolutely necessary and, if so, to consult with the mother as well as with her own physician and pediatrician to determine the best option for a breastfeeding mother. This statement also suggests that if there is any concern about a particular drug a mother might need to take, physicians can instruct mothers to take the drug immediately after breastfeeding or just before the infant is expected to sleep for several hours.[21]

There is of course always a legitimate reason for concern regarding medications that can be passed to the infant through the mother's milk, and most physicians would agree it is best to avoid medications that are not absolutely necessary. However, breastfeeding experts have noted that too often breastfeeding is unnecessarily disrupted because physicians do not take the time to investigate the safety of the drug they are prescribing. Often times, even if a drug is deemed dangerous to the infant, physicians can find safer alternatives if they consult specialized sources such as Hale's reference. As suggested by the story told above, when health-care practitioners do not take the time to seek out accurate information, they often base their recommendations on guesses or assumptions. In this mother's story, for instance, there is nothing in the available literature to suggest that weaning for twenty-four hours after ingesting one dose of Vicodin was necessary; if the mother and physician had wanted to be on the safe side, ceasing breastfeeding for six to eight hours probably would have been sufficient to make sure the drug was out of the mother's system, and this shorter period of cessation might have made it easier for the mother to resume the breastfeeding relationship. Furthermore, and more important, if breastfeeding had been considered an important part of the health-care situation from the beginning, the physician would have presented the mother with some other options. If she had known at the outset that other medications were available, the mother might have selected a weaker one that would have posed even less possible risk to the nursing infant. Instead, this mother was placed in a situation that seemed to provide her with only one option. This situation ultimately made it impossible for this mother to continue breastfeeding.

In addition to stories of faulty medical advice that interfered with breast-feeding, another important type of story that research participants tell involves situations in which the mother seemed to have no access to any type of breast-feeding advice at a time when she really needed it. For instance, one particularly troubling story came from a focus-group participant, Danielle, who had switched to the bottle because she felt her newborn was starving. This mother said early in the conversation, "I always knew that I would breastfeed." But, in her words, "life always hands you something that you're not really planning for." As her story unfolded, this mother continued to talk about her experience as a disappointment. For instance, she responded as follows to another mother who had commented that the choice to breastfeed had been taken away from her: "The same way that it was taken away from you, you weren't able to breastfeed. I couldn't also breastfeed her. She wouldn't latch on. She wouldn't, she just decided that it wasn't for her. It was her decision."

The focus groups turned up numerous stories similar to this one—situations in which mothers felt they were unable to breastfeed as long as they had wanted. But what makes this particular story especially remarkable is that later in the conversation, it became clear that this woman had stopped breast-feeding when her infant was only four days old: "Yes, she was four days old before we were finally, like, this baby is starving—she's not eating. And so we just had to switch to formula."

Most breastfeeding experts today would agree that, especially for a first-time mother, it is not uncommon for a mother's milk to take four to five days before it completely "comes in."[22] In fact, newborns really do not need to consume large amounts of milk in their first few days, so most likely, if this woman had waited another day or two, her milk supply would have increased, and when that happened, the baby would have started latching and sucking more vigorously. The fact that this woman determined on day 4 that her baby could not latch is another clear example of a breastfeeding problem that could have been easily remedied if this woman had had access to a knowledgeable health care professional who valued breastfeeding and knew how to help the woman accurately interpret the signs being communicated by her own body and that of her infant.

One of the doulas interviewed, Trisha, commented that the issue of milk "coming in" is one on which she repeatedly has to educate mothers and health-care professionals. As she said: "I've had to explain and re-explain and then know that it's going in one ear and out the other of some mothers because, you know, they were told that until your milk, quote, comes in, there's nothing there. You're going to starve them. You know, they don't understand the whole process. And so, it's just a battle. . . . You still have some old school nurses out there who insist that those babies need to be given water and sugar water and this and that."

This potential for problematic advice in the hospital environment is compounded by the fact that women in the United States often attempt breastfeeding for the first time with few mental pictures of others who have breastfed babies and, therefore, with no point of reference to indicate what breastfeeding is supposed to look like and how the breastfed baby is supposed to act. The importance of support from other women is widely acknowledged in the public-health literature. For instance, one team of researchers studied the infant-feeding experiences of a small sample of low-income mothers in the United Kingdom and found that even though all sixteen mothers in the study had expressed a desire to breastfeed while they were pregnant, they also expressed a strong expectation that they would fail. In many cases, these researchers found, this expectation of failure was borne out when the mothers tried breastfeeding in the first few days after birth: "The participants' interpretations of what happened when they 'tried to succeed' suggests again that they struggle from within a culture that undermines breast feeding or at least does not expect success."[23] Studies in the United States also provide quantitative and qualitative data to document this phenomenon. Especially when they focus on mothers from demographic groups with lower breastfeeding rates, such studies document high rates of breastfeeding attrition during the first several weeks after birth, suggesting a significant gap between mothers' intentions during pregnancy and their actual experiences with breastfeeding after the baby is born.[24] These studies all conclude that most of the mothers who discontinued breastfeeding earlier than they had planned did so for reasons that could have been corrected by a knowledgeable lactation consultant, but mothers did not have access to such breastfeeding support after they left the hospital. Some studies have also taken a closer look at the interpersonal dynamics that shape a mother's infant-feeding experience, showing how various sources of information, including grandmothers and other relatives and also official sources such as WIC, confront mothers with contradictory messages about infant feeding and interact in complex ways with the messages that mothers receive from health-care practitioners to shape their actual experiences with infant feeding.[25] Because such studies have identified major gaps and conflicts among these various information sources, they further illuminate the reasons why gaps might exist between a mother's stated intentions during pregnancy and her actual experience after birth.[26]

My interview data reinforce the findings that are reported in these public-health studies and allow us to closely examine, as a uniquely rhetorical problem, situations in which breastfeeding fails due to faulty medical advice. Recalling the lines from Plato's dialogue cited in the epigraph to this book, when we hear the interviewees' stories, we cannot help but be awakened to the centrality of rhetoric to aspects of life such as infant feeding that are subject to medical expertise and intervention. From a rhetorical perspective, the general lack of a cultural reference point converges with the conflicting messages that women often receive in medical settings. These circumstances circumscribe what the breastfeeding body can do and make it even more difficult to follow the AAP's recommendation to breastfeed for at least one year.

As interviewee Sharon observed, the long-standing tendency for women to see far more examples of bottle-feeding mothers than breastfeeding mothers often leads breastfeeding women to doubt the capabilities of their own bodies: "Most people have enough milk," but "most people think they don't have enough milk, . . . so perceived insufficient milk is a big problem." She elaborated on the subject, claiming that women's doubts about their bodies can ultimately interfere with lactation itself: "It's a leap of faith to think that your body can nourish a baby; . . . often times, the mom's insecurities will lead to supplementation and ultimate weaning."

As postpartum doula Diane observed, pregnant women often take a breast-feeding class offered by the hospital where they plan to give birth. However, this in itself is not enough to make breastfeeding seem like a normal activity because many women "grew up without seeing enough women breastfeeding, so we're not internalizing the images of breastfeeding." Michelle, a La Leche League leader, echoed Diane, asserting that our "culture has set a lot of women up [to fail] at breastfeeding" because expectations that infants should adopt regular sleep patterns and admonitions against "pacifying the baby with the breast" are based on behaviors more typical of bottle-fed than breastfed babies.

Examples from the focus groups abound. Time and time again, mothers told stories from their own experiences or someone else they knew in which breastfeeding "didn't work out." The following are just a few examples:

"I'm thinking about giving up because I'm not producing enough milk." (Alexia)

"Yes, my first son—I breastfed for eight weeks. And it was like water. Nothing came out. My child was starving and I was nineteen. No patience. So I just popped a bottle in his mouth and he was happy then." (Tracy)

"And another reason why it wouldn't work out is because, after I had her, I got sick—postpartum depression—and I didn't eat a lot, so I lost a lot of weight. And I lost a lot of milk." (Jessica)

"My mom wasn't able to breastfeed. She had milk, but it wouldn't, like, come out. Something was wrong in that area. So she wasn't able to breastfeed, but she wanted to." (Rebecca)

As these quotations suggest, the expectation of breastfeeding failure is so great that often there is no perceived need for an explanation. And when an explanation is provided, the blame is frequently placed on a defect in the mother's own body. In fact, quite often in cases like these, the inability to breastfeed is actually caused by material circumstances beyond the mothers' control, even though mothers talk about it as a physical incapacity or a limitation of their own bodies. The situations these women describe can lead to serious breastfeeding problems, and whether these problems are imagined or real, they can lead the mother to believe that it is necessary to wean from breast to bottle, even if weaning is not medically warranted, and even if she does not want to do it. In theoretical terms, then, breastfeeding advocates' and mothers' remarks about the ways in which health-care practitioners, or even friends and relatives, can undermine breastfeeding success offer an example of disciplinary rhetoric circumscribing what a woman's body is able to achieve. Even if she is told that she should breastfeed for at least a year, the institutional practice of offering unnecessary supplements or unnecessarily advising a mother to wean, as well as cultural perceptions based on the model of bottle-fed babies, can make it difficult or impossible to do so. As their remarks indicate, even if women today are educated in breastfeeding techniques and the benefits of breastfeeding, they often receive conflicting advice from either medical authorities or friends and relatives that undermines successful breastfeeding, literally making their bodies unable to lactate successfully. This is the larger framework in which women attempt breastfeeding today. This expectation of failure has been widely documented in the public-health and medical sociology literature. Previous research has demonstrated that expectation of breastfeeding failure is widespread, especially among low-income mothers and ethnic minorities.[27] Multiple studies have also indicated a wide gap between mothers' intentions to breastfeed and actual breastfeeding rates.[28]

"Bucking the System"

Although it is important to keep documenting and analyzing the experiences of women who feel they have failed at breastfeeding, it is also important to take a close look at the rhetorical dimensions of situations in which women succeed at breastfeeding in spite of cultural situations that set them up to fail. What are the rhetorical strategies that women use to overcome the many obstacles to breastfeeding success that exist in our culture, and what might we learn about possibilities for large-scale change from closely examining these strategies? Because the disciplinary rhetorics that surround breastfeeding as an embodied practice often make breastfeeding impossible even as they recommend it as the ideal feeding method, mothers who are successful at breastfeeding often define their experiences in terms of resistance. But their stories also show how it is possible to succeed despite problematic circumstances, and, as such, they suggest how we might envision a future that is more truly supportive of breastfeeding success.

As suggested by the epigraph to this chapter, acting in the context of disciplinary rhetoric entails a certain degree of risk, especially when that action involves direct questioning of a medical authority. Despite this difficulty, however, the women I interviewed over the last decade have told numerous stories in which they or someone else they knew had asserted their own authority in the context of disciplinary rhetorics that interfere with breastfeeding. Such actions often involved resisting faulty medical advice or continuing to breastfeed even when friends and relatives discouraged it. In the words of one La Leche League leader, "Kim," to breastfeed a baby in our society a woman has to "buck the system." Reflecting this observation, multiple women in my study have reported instances in which they actively exercised some degree of choice among the competing discourses that form the framework of meaning established by the disciplinary rhetorics of breastfeeding, and if they had not been aware of the ability to make such choices, they would have had to give up breastfeeding.

In my initial interviews with breastfeeding advocates, the rhetorical agency that women enacted often took the form of directly challenging something they had heard a physician say. For instance, the lactation consultant Sharon recounted how she had used the 1997 AAP policy statement to educate the physicians in her hospital and even to bolster her credibility in disagreements with such physicians: "I have made stacks of copies [of the 1997 statement] and put them in the resident lounge, I have slipped one under the door of our chief perinatalogist when he differed with me on a certain point. . . . There was an instance where I was telling a mom that, for the most part, breast milk is all the baby needs for the first six months, and there was a doctor behind the curtain, who then came around the curtain, and he said 'but that may not be true for all babies; check with the baby's doctor on that,' and I gave him a copy [of the 1997 statement]."

In contrast to Sharon's reliance on the AAP policy statement to challenge physicians' authority, some of the breastfeeding advocates from this initial set of interviews emphasized the unique perspective that the distinctly nonmedical knowledge of an organization such as La Leche League provides to breastfeeding women. In fact, many of these interviewees claimed that their own needs for alternatives to mainstream medical discourse when they began breastfeeding led them to become La Leche League leaders or lactation consultants in the first place.

For instance, according to Janet, a board-certified lactation consultant and La Leche League leader, she first attended La Leche League when her first daughter was young because it offered her an alternative way to read her body and understand the breastfeeding relationship, allowing her to reject the emphasis on scheduled feedings that she had learned through mainstream medical discourse: "I enjoyed the information and support that I got. Among other things, I needed to hear that I didn't have to let babies cry in order to wait a certain number of hours between feedings, so we had a lot less crying at our house when I started going to meetings, and I started to trust myself a little more as a mother instead of just coming more from my nursing background of doing things on a schedule." Similarly, Kim, a La Leche League leader, described the role of La Leche League as filling in the gaps in mainstream medical practice—providing the "practical stuff that women need, the actual nuts and bolts of how the relationship works and what to do when there's problems."

Providing a more specific example, Jackie, also a La Leche League leader, tells the story of one woman who had consulted her regarding a physician's recommendation for treatment of a thyroid problem. According to Jackie, this woman eventually opted for the treatment that preserved the breastfeeding relationship, even though this choice meant that she had to question the physician's initial recommendations:

> "I know one woman who was told she needed to do the radioactive treatment to kill off her thyroid gland because she was hyperthyroid, and to do that . . . she would have to wean her baby for . . . a week or ten days. And she said, 'I don't want to do that. What else can we do?' And the doctor said, 'Oh, well, this is the only way to treat the problem other than surgical removal of your thyroid gland.'. . . She said, 'When I look at my options, this is a minor surgical procedure, that's going to have a two-hour separation between me and my baby, versus something that's going to require me to wean for . . . fourteen days.'. . . She opted for the surgical removal of her thyroid rather than killing it off with a radioactive drug."

In this case, it was the willingness of a woman to question a physician's recommendations directly that allowed her to continue breastfeeding. Along these lines, many of the breastfeeding advocates interviewed have noted that their job is not only to provide alternative information but also to empower women so that they will feel confident enough to ask the kinds of questions that will solicit such information from their physicians. As Sharon said, an important part of her job is "to give [mothers] the confidence that they can provide enough milk for the baby, and be assertive for themselves when deal-ing with health professionals." Of course, La Leche League perpetuates its own forms of disciplinary rhetorics, some of which have discouraged moth-ers from working outside the home and have idealized motherhood in ways that make feminist scholars understandably uncomfortable.[29] Thus, La Leche League cannot be understood as simply a source of empowerment. Nonethe-less, in the stories that many research participants have told, La Leche League does seem to serve as an important source of alternative information for moth-ers who seek a counterdiscourse in situations in which mainstream medical advice would otherwise thwart breastfeeding.

In the more recent interviews, a Texas mother, Grace, told a story in which her newborn had to be hospitalized for a medical condition requiring surgery. Although she was advised to stop nursing, she kept up the breastfeeding rela-tionship by pumping for seventy-two hours while her baby was hospitalized:

> "They said put the crib, you know, up at an angle. Let her sleep upright. And get her on formula. And I was, like, you know, I've got an instinct that says her body's not lacking in formula. So, we just kept on with the nurs-ing. And that's what they had explained to me, as long as I'm pumping, I wasn't going to dry up, and that was my fear. And so I just kept pumping and the nurses would feed her. And so we were probably, she was probably in the hospital maybe three days. So it was probably seventy-two hours, I guess."

In this mother's case, it was her relationship with the midwives who had delivered her baby in a birthing center that allowed her to resist the medical advice to wean. As she said:

> "So like twenty-four hours before the surgery, you can't eat. And so every time she'd see me in the room she would cry. And then that would make me produce more milk, and I got a breast infection, ran a 104 fever. So I was sick. But [the midwives], . . . even though we were in Dallas and they were in Austin, we were still communicating. . . . The midwives said you got to get a pump and pump the milk. And so, I would pump the milk, but still they wouldn't let me nurse her because they wanted to monitor how much food she was eating. So we'd have to pump it, and then they would put it in a bottle. Because I was, like, I don't want her to have for-mula. And even my doctors told me when she was spitting up, 'Oh, she's allergic to your breast milk. You need to get her on formula.'"

Stories such as these illustrate how rhetorical agency, defined as negotia-tion among competing alternative discourses, grants individuals some ability to reject discursive elements that they find problematic. Such accounts of resis-tance have precedents in previous communication scholarship. For instance, in her study of a 1987 Massachusetts mandate requiring insurance companies to cover infertility treatments, Elizabeth C. Britt invokes the concept of the double bind to explain "both how discourses create spaces within which individuals act and how individuals act within these spaces."[30] Based on her research, Britt argues that the individual can exercise some degree of agency by choosing among the alternatives offered by double binds: "The individual is not a passive subject of biopower but makes decisions and takes actions . . . . Far from being autonomous agents, individuals nevertheless make choices between competing alternatives."[31] In his study of the discourses of HIV testing, J. Blake Scott echoes Britt's findings, asserting that the individual examined in his study is "not a docile body straightforwardly shaped by the testing program's disciplinary rhetorics" but is "conditioned by the national pedagogy, interpersonal relationships, and cultural norms."[32]

Although these communication scholars stress that individuals can exercise some choice among competing discourses, they also remind us that subjects cannot necessarily escape such discourses. For instance, Britt concludes that some women in her study felt "empowered by working themselves out of double binds."[33] But Britt ultimately adopts a cautious stance toward such agency and empowerment, noting that choosing among the alternatives they appear to offer does not necessarily resolve double binds and that some double binds might be entrenched in our culture to such an extent that they are nearly impossible for individuals to resolve.[34] Along similar lines, Scott concludes that subjects of HIV testing discourse might have some ability to "negotiate the alternative notions of risk" conveyed in such discourse, but that it is hard to know how much negotiation will be possible in any given situation.[35]

These discussions of rhetorical agency and its limitations raise important questions about how to interpret the acts of resistance that many of the interviewees quoted have described. On the one hand, these discussions make clear that the rhetorical agency exerted by women who continue breastfeeding in spite of conflicting messages from health-care authorities or the culture at large cannot be understood simply as strategic, subject-centered language use that enables them to escape the grid of meaning established by disciplinary rhetoric. But on the other hand, if we acknowledge the extent to which this grid of meaning continues to circumscribe their actions, it is not clear whether the actions that interviewees describe truly count as resistance. Whether they appeal to alternative discourses within medicine, such as the AAP policy statement, to nonmedical discourses such as information from La Leche League, or even to friends and family members, it could be argued that the alternative discourses these women marshal are simply alternative forms of disciplinary rhetoric. Extending this line of reasoning, one might argue that the women are not really subverting the disciplinary power that circumscribes the breastfeeding experience but rather are choosing among several preexisting subject positions made available to them within its framework. More important, in light of the goal of developing a rhetorical understanding of breastfeeding, it is not clear whether these women's individual acts of resistance have any far-reaching effects that will change the larger framework of disciplinary rhetorics in ways that will make breastfeeding easier for other women.

Foucault offers insight into questions such as these in his assertion that, even though resistant acts "can only exist in the strategic field of power relations," such acts do not have to be understood as just "a reaction or rebound, forming with respect to the basic domination an underside that is in the end always passive, doomed to perpetual defeat."[36] In other words, Foucault suggests, it might be possible to disrupt disciplinary power even without escaping its grip. The women interviewed suggest how this type of disruption might be possible when they discuss more specifically the relationships between their rhetorical agency and the effects of the resistance that this agency allows. Specifically, in these discussions we begin to see that resistance might initially involve a form of rhetorical agency in which subjects simply occupy preexisting subject positions. But the effects of this agency—the acts of resistance—can disrupt the sense established by disciplinary rhetoric, exceeding the boundaries of these subject positions in unpredictable ways.

Some of the most striking examples that interviewees have offered in this regard are those that include instances in which they shocked medical authorities, friends, or acquaintances by defying preconceived notions of what women's bodies are capable of doing. For instance, Karen, a board-certified lactation consultant in a large suburban hospital, talked about nursing twins several years ago and repeatedly having to address the astonishment of health-care professionals and others who did not believe this act should have been possible: "I have twins, and, of course, everyone said, 'well, you're not gonna breastfeed twins, are you?' And so I had a really nice lady, a lactation consultant; . . . she said, 'you know what, tell them you have two breasts just in case you have two babies,' and, so, I've hung onto that ever since."

As another example, Ellen, a La Leche League leader, talked about her earlier experience of breastfeeding a premature baby. Because premature babies are typically not able to breastfeed directly, a mother has to pump breast milk and feed it to the baby through a feeding tube. As Ellen's remarks make clear, this is not something that many mothers had done at that time, and part of what made it possible for her is that she had the support of a lactation consultant in the hospital where she and her baby were staying:

"In looking back on it now, what I did with a preemie I guess is pretty rare. There aren't very many preemies who successfully breastfeed . . . but, you know, I never got that perception when I was doing it. I was just pumping, and you know, I just kept pumping. I was, like, what else am I gonna do? . . . I had nothing to do except get this baby home, and that was my goal. And, you know, even once in a while the doctor would come in and say, 'I'm very impressed that you're still keeping up with this. Most moms give up by now.'. . . And the lactation consultant there was very helpful, and the nurses were very helpful and encouraging. And so, I think that made a world of difference, knowing that there was that support system there."

As we see in these accounts, interviewees still depend on the kind of rhetorical negotiation among competing alternatives within the grid of meaning established by disciplinary rhetoric that could be construed as the occupation of preexisting subject positions. Specifically, in both accounts the women emphasize that they needed the support of someone like a La Leche League leader or lactation consultant to enable them to carry out the actions they consider resistant. But because these accounts refer specifically to the reactions of other people who are implicated in the grid of meaning established by disciplinary rhetoric, we also begin to see how this grid might be disrupted when subjects perform acts that this grid had previously defined as impossible. If one recalls that disciplinary rhetorics define what individuals can do as well as what they should do, these women can be seen as disrupting sense by accomplishing things that disciplinary rhetorics dictated they could not do. The surprised reactions of bystanders including medical authorities, friends, and relatives can be read as an indication of the potential for such disruption.

Although it confronts a set of issues different from those we have addressed so far, the issue of nursing in public places offers another useful example of the nuances of this relationship between rhetorical agency and resistance. Although many states now have laws that explicitly protect a woman's right to breastfeed in public, it is far from being accepted as a normal activity in our society as a whole, and it is something that many women still do not feel comfortable doing, and probably for good reason. On November 10, 2003, a Burger King employee at an Orem, Utah, restaurant asked a customer who was breastfeeding her baby to leave. The employee's request was reportedly a response to the remarks of another customer who claimed to feel uncomfortable with the mother's public breastfeeding. Burger King later issued an official apology.[37] More recently, on June 14, 2007, something similar happened at an Applebee's restaurant in Lexington, Kentucky, when a mother was asked to stop nursing her seven-month-old baby because other customers had complained to the manager.[38]

Similar stories about mothers being chastised for public breastfeeding recur in the news periodically—so much so that they hardly garner much attention anymore, unless they reach the level of legal action or spark mothers to call for a "nurse-in" or engage in other types of activism. Because of these conflicting attitudes about public breastfeeding in our society, many women feel uncomfortable with public breastfeeding, even if they know it is legally protected, and if they do not personally disapprove of others doing it. The feelings of discomfort can be especially intense for the first-time mother who has not breastfed in public before. Thus, more than one interviewee explicitly mentioned that a La Leche League meeting can be a good place to prepare a woman for her first experience with public nursing. As Diane, a postpartum doula, said: "It's kind of a culture shock when you walk into a La Leche League meeting and see all these breastfeeding mothers, and you've never seen even one in your life, and all of a sudden you've got a room full of them, you know, one nursing a baby and a toddler on the other side."

Lisa, a La Leche League leader, explains, however, that despite this preparation, a woman is still on her own the first time she nurses in public outside of a League meeting: a La Leche meeting "is a good place to go over that particular wall. And it is, . . . like a wall when you first breastfeed in public, you know, you think all eyes are on you, you feel like you're thirteen, and so that can be a good place to come."

As we see in the example of public nursing, resistance is not just a question of an individual selecting bits and pieces from various competing discourses. By consulting La Leche League, which resists mainstream medical discourse as well as broadly accepted social and cultural norms, the woman is empowered to resist the cultural norm that forbids public breastfeeding, but the ultimate effect of her choice is not scripted in the predefined subject position she selects. Specifically, at the moment she actually breastfeeds in public by herself for the first time, a woman is forced to act in a space where the counterdiscourse of La Leche League is not that which prevails. It is at this moment, I would argue, she has the potential to disrupt sense.

As expressed by Michel de Certeau, "the users of social codes turn them into metaphors and ellipses of their own quests."[39] Certeau compares the individual use of social codes to "the rules of meter and rhyme for poets of earlier times: a body of constraints stimulating new discoveries, a set of rules with which improvisation plays."[40] In other words, the impetus to resist might start with an action that could be construed as simply occupying a pre-existing subject position (or use of a pre-existing "social code" in Certeau's terms): identifying oneself as aligned with the cultural norms of La Leche League, rather than with mainstream cultural norms, which do not widely condone public nursing. However, when one considers the moment at which a woman first attempts nursing in a public space outside of a La Leche League meeting, the occupation of pre-existing subject positions is no longer an adequate explanation of her actions; the ultimate effect of asserting rhetorical agency in this type of situation is something more than the sense, or meaning, made possible by disciplinary rhetoric's grid of meaning, because the effect of overcoming "the wall" when a mother breastfeeds in public for the first time is unknown. Whereas she knows she will be safe violating this cultural norm in the safe space of a La Leche League meeting, she does not know what she will face when she breastfeeds for the first time in a shopping mall, restaurant, or other public space.

Participants in the focus groups offered further stories to illustrate this phenomenon. A few participants told stories about defiantly nursing in public, even in situations or places where this act was obviously not deemed acceptable. As Nancy said: "I went almost a full year nursing my daughter without ever seeing anybody else nursing in public. I was at Oklahoma City at the mall with some of my friends and there was a woman there nursing her child. And I said, 'Oh my gosh!' She is the only other woman I have ever seen since [my baby] was born—besides myself—nursing in public. So I wondered how many looks I really was getting but not paying attention to. Because I tried to tune it out."

The language that participants used to recount such experiences often conveyed a sense of personal rights and freedom or adopted a critical stance toward U.S. sexual norms. Most study participants talked about social disapproval of public breastfeeding in rather abstract terms—something they imagined but never directly encountered. However, in a few examples, mothers reported being verbally harassed for breastfeeding in public, even though Texas does have a law that explicitly protects a woman's rights to do this. In fact, the same focus-group participant, Nancy, also told a story in which she continued nursing her infant even while being verbally harassed: "I nursed my daughter under a blanket pretty much wherever you can imagine—restaurants, my brother's awards assembly. We were in the middle of a row and it would have been so disruptive to take her out, so I just covered her up and, of course, most people didn't notice. I did have this eighteen-year-old kid slurp behind me, which really annoyed me. I wanted to turn around and smack him. But it was really all I could do not to just throw an arm [gestures hitting a person behind her]."

In an even more troubling story, one focus-group participant, Julie, told of feeling harassed while she breastfed her newborn in her own car. Although the act was clearly visible to interested bystanders, it is difficult to define this act as public by any stretch of the imagination. Julie told the story as follows: "I covered. I did it for the first time a few days ago. And a guy was standing nearby— I was in my car, my boyfriend was in the store—and I covered myself up. And I was being very discreet. And I'm all trying to cover myself up [demonstrates]. And he was just standing there watching me breastfeed. And I'm, like, [surprised look]. So I take her off and he goes back inside and I fix up and I'm, like, 'Man, screw this, get me a bottle.' I was very embarrassed and I felt very uncomfortable." When asked for further clarification, it became clear that the man was simply walking by when he stopped and stared at this mother: "Yeah, he was just walking by, and he was just standing there watching me, and I was, like, trying to hide myself [imitates sinking in her seat]."

Although it might be easy from an outside perspective to judge that this man was clearly in the wrong and that the woman should have ignored him and continued to breastfeed, as is her right, we cannot ignore the fact that she felt harassed. This was a first-time mother with a baby who was two weeks old at the time of participation in the focus group. The harassment that she reportedly experienced for public breastfeeding occurred while she was in her own parked car.

As these various stories of public breastfeeding illustrate, the forms of resistance described in this section involve rhetorical agency, but they also involve a moment when the subject does more than just select among competing alternatives within the disciplinary grid—a moment when the subject suggests that her actions disrupt the sense of this grid, or at least have the potential to do so. And this moment entails a certain degree of personal risk: even when laws are in place to protect the act of public breastfeeding, the outcome of enacting this personal right is not guaranteed. To understand further this potential for disruption and how it might contribute to the long-term effects of resistance, it helps to expand our thinking beyond the isolated moment or event that each woman describes. Scott calls for this type of expansion in his stipulation that the "process of subject formation . . . cannot be located in a discrete event or set of events, and cannot simply be viewed as the product of that event's discourse or interaction between rhetorical agents."[41] In other words, the rhetorical agency and acts of resistance described by the focus-group participants must not be reduced to individual acts with distinct beginning and end points, but rather must be understood as, at least potentially, having implications that extend beyond the individual events or acts they describe.

Although the present study is not equipped to track systematically the long-term effects of resistant acts in precisely the manner that this expanded view requires, the potential for long-term disruption of sense is at least suggested in one interviewee's suggestion that as infant-feeding norms gradually change, the "feats" women accomplish might come to be seen as less remarkable. Specifically, Jackie, a La Leche League leader, described an instance in which she challenged medical perceptions about what her body should be capable of doing: "When my second one was born ten and a half years ago, one of the nurses asked me, right after he was born—I had him latched on—she said 'Wow you're a pro at this, when was the last time you nursed?' and I glanced at the clock and said 'Oh, about twelve hours ago.'" And that absolutely stunned them, that I had nursed through a pregnancy. . . . That was quite an outrageous thing for them to be confronted with because I know I wasn't the first woman to do that, but I was the first one to admit it."

In this description of an instance in which she defied medical perceptions of what is possible, Jackie's account resembles those of other interviewees. But Jackie also went on to explain that, in her opinion, this same act is now less likely to be seen as remarkable because more health-care practitioners have encountered something like it: "And now you find more nurses who know it's OK to nurse through a pregnancy, or they'll talk about, 'Yeah, there was a mom in here, and she was nursing a newborn on one side and her eighteen-month-old nursing on the other side at the same time, and wasn't that sweet,' rather than, 'I can't believe the doctor allowed that.'"

Jackie's remarks suggest how the individual resistant acts that other interviewees describe might over time have a profound impact in the lines of sense established by disciplinary rhetoric. Although Jackie's remarks pertain to an encounter with medical authorities, it is easy to imagine that these remarks might apply to the issue of public breastfeeding as well—that is, we might speculate that if enough women continue to disrupt sense by violating cultural norms that forbid public breastfeeding, these norms will eventually change. And, in fact, several participants in the focus groups felt that public breastfeeding is becoming more acceptable, even if they did not personally condone it or would not feel comfortable doing it themselves. The following quotes from focus-group participants provide examples:

> "When I was a child, women were kind of ashamed to breastfeed in front of people. Nowadays, they don't care much." (Mark)

> "Plus, wasn't breastfeeding in public looked down upon back then? Because they were all about decency and, like, you don't do that in public. That was just rude." (Theresa)

> "Society is a lot more open to it now. You can see a woman breastfeeding on an airplane or in a restaurant, or, you know, some people, some women, they still go in the bathroom stall and do it. And some people just don't care—they lift up their shirt and there you go. And, yeah, society has changed their opinions on it. Society is a lot more comfortable with it now. Society as a whole has changed as far as decency, as far as to what's decent and what's not. . . . I think the whole opinion in society has helped it push along and get to where it is now rather than, opposed to how it was back in the sixties and seventies." (Rebecca)

Of course, we must acknowledge that these outcomes are only possibilities, not guarantees; just as sense can be disrupted through individual acts of resistance, it can be put back into place through new forms of disciplinary rhetoric that aim to restrict further what is possible and permissible—a point that is poignantly expressed in the stories of women who experience harassment when breastfeeding in public. Until further research is done on this subject, we cannot know which of these outcomes will prevail in the case of resistance to the disciplinary rhetorics of breastfeeding.

Making Breastfeeding Possible

Reinforcing the findings of previous communication research, the focus-group data presented suggest that the multiplicity of breastfeeding discourse makes resistance possible because it allows women some ability to determine the outcome of their own breastfeeding experiences by actively negotiating among the competing messages they receive from friends, relatives, the media, and health-care professionals. However, it also reinforces the idea that this ability to choose has limits. More than one of the women I have interviewed over the last decade has expressed that her choice to breastfeed was taken away, and many of these women, particularly in the focus groups, had described situations in which breastfeeding was literally made impossible because they lacked access to a knowledgeable health-care professional or, in the most unfortunate cases, because they were given incorrect medical advice that caused them to wean.

In addition to affirming these observations of previous research, analysis of the focus-group data has shed further light on a question that we continue to face as communication researchers: how can we account for some individuals' abilities to resist disciplinary rhetoric without resorting to understandings that might oversimplify the situations these individuals face or underestimate the difficulties they encounter? In response to this question, I have demonstrated that although the forms of resistance many interviewees have described might be understood as the acting out of subject positions that pre-exist their actions, not all of the effects of these resistant acts are contained within the scripts that define such positions. In fact, some of the acts of resistance that interviewees have described entail reading and writing their bodies into the disciplinary grid in ways that disrupt the sense of this grid. In these examples, it is not only literate practices but also physical actions and ways of using the body (especially those that threaten the social order by doing things deemed impossible or violating cultural norms) that become integral to understanding how individuals resist the authority of powerful institutional discourses.

In a culture in which mothers are often assigned primary responsibility for their infants' health and well-being, regardless of whether the prevailing discourse at a given historical moment privileges breast or bottle-feeding, conversations about rhetorical agency and resistance in the face of the ideological force of medical discourse have implications that extend beyond academic conversations. Just as placing too much emphasis on the ideological force of such discourses can obscure individuals' abilities to resist such force, placing too much emphasis on the ability to resist might lead us to ignore the dangers and difficulties people can encounter in disobeying medical authority or violating cultural norms. Such an emphasis might be especially risky if it fuels the cultural tendency to assign women too much blame for the difficulties they can encounter in aspects of life such as infant feeding and thus overlooks the need for larger social, cultural, and institutional changes that would make breastfeeding more acceptable.

For this reason, the findings we have presented should be of interest to scholars participating in the effort to develop a feminist discourse of breastfeeding. Yet the conflicts in the messages that today's mothers are hearing about breastfeeding have gone largely unnoticed in current feminist critiques of the medical community's recent enthusiasm about breastfeeding. Instead, feminist scholars tend to emphasize the "axiomatic" nature of medicine's current encouragement of breastfeeding.[42] Generalizations such as these overlook the numerous conflicts that still exist with regard to infant-feeding advice delivered in the context of medical practice.

Admittedly, my interview research has been qualitative in nature, and thus I have no basis for claiming these women's experiences are universal. However, the sample of women involved in this research has been developed according to sound principles of sample selection. As such, the sample has become increasingly diverse over time. And at each step along the way, I have sought to extend the sample in a manner that would force me to question the conclusions I was starting to draw from the previous sample. Although this sampling approach cannot guarantee that my results can be generalized to the whole U.S. population, it does minimize the likelihood that my findings are entirely idiosyncratic or confined to the individuals who participated in this study. Thus, even if they are not universal, the stories told here and the conclusions drawn about these stories should be taken seriously—they have happened time and time again, and they persist across the various demographic boundaries that public-health scholars typically use to categorize the factors that influence women's infant-feeding decisions. Furthermore, I would argue, some events deserve critical attention even if they only happen one time. For instance, when we hear stories in which a woman has been incorrectly advised that she needed to wean, has been given advice that directly interferes with successful lactation, or has been harassed for breastfeeding in public, we need to take such stories seriously whether they represent one occurrence or one hundred.

As we continue to study breastfeeding from various disciplinary perspectives, we need to keep in mind the theoretical and practical realities we have reviewed. If we continue to resist the tendency to assign too much responsibility to individuals or to institutions, we can continue finding new and better ways to acknowledge rhetorical agency and resistance without using this awareness to blame individuals for complex social problems. In particular, we need more studies of the long-term effects of rhetorical agency and resistance as they play out in the unique context of infant feeding, so that we can gain a more precise understanding of the limitations as well as the possibilities inherent in them. In the realm of medical practice, we need to continue to place more emphasis on educating health-care professionals on the realities of breastfeeding practice and making them better at providing advice to mothers who ask for it. Continuing to tout the health benefits of breastfeeding is not enough. Clearly, mothers have internalized the message that they should breastfeed, but as a society we all need more reminders that most women can do it.

6

....

Feminism, Rhetoric, and Breastfeeding

Some Concluding Remarks

In an August 29, 2008, interview with *People* magazine, vice-presidential candidate Sarah Palin was asked how she could handle running for vice president while being a mother of five children, one of whom was still an infant. Palin started with her usual reply about the many challenges she had faced, but on this occasion she added some interesting language: "What I've had to do, though, is in the middle of the night, put down the Blackberries and pick up the breast pump."[1] That single reference to the breast pump circulated briefly through the media but then quickly vanished. Other than that one fleeting reference to a breast pump, the popular media never portrayed Palin having anything to do with feeding her baby. Palin was depicted as a super mom, hated by some, revered by others. But apparently, at least in the public view, she was able to breastfeed without ever stopping her political activity for a moment, either to pump milk, nurse the baby, or wipe spit-up milk from her expensive suit.

Palin's media image perpetuated the idea of the mom who can have a baby and go back to work the next day. Although her devoted followers touted her accomplishments as evidence that today's woman can "have it all," her many critics shuddered to think that her example would be used as further justification for why we need not worry about issues such as parental leave, health care, and work–family balance.[2] If Sarah can do it without any help from the state, why can't we all? Indeed one of the most troubling aspects of the brief time that Palin as vice-presidential candidate enjoyed in the media spotlight was that it perpetuated the idea of good motherhood as clean,

130

seamless, sanitary, and, perhaps most important, as not interfering with any-one else's business. As long as a woman is part of a nuclear family that includes a dear husband willing to pitch in and help, she can effortlessly combine career success with a happy family of breastfed children, and she can still look good while she does it—disembodied mothering, we might call it.

Of course, there is much more feminist analysis that could be done on Sarah Palin as a rhetorical phenomenon. But my main concern is that the media spotlight that exposed Palin as a vice-presidential candidate provides a concrete example of what could otherwise be dismissed as a purely theoretical problem: the one voice that has been barely audible amid the cacophony of discourses that circulate around breastfeeding in the early twenty-first-century United States, as Bernice L. Hausman has astutely observed, is a feminist voice, or in Hausman's words, a "feminist discourse" of breastfeeding.[3] This absence is unfortunate, as Hausman says, because "lactating women lack a feminist discourse to frame their experience, both as embodied mothers and as social beings who interact with others in a society that discourages their use of their bodies to feed their infants."[4] Thus, we are left with a set of options that do not seem terribly appealing. On the one hand, we have the Sarah Palins of the world, whipping out the breast pump in the middle of the night and seeming to engage in motherhood, and even breastfeeding, without any visible evidence of embodiment whatsoever. On the other hand, we have the rest of us, strug-gling to make sense of infant feeding in a way that feels all too embodied in all too many ways. Indeed, when we hear women tell their own stories about their infant-feeding experiences, it is all about the bodies. It is about bodies that work or do not work, bodies that get scrutinized for public behavior that some believe should be done in private, bodies that are judged as either pure or contaminated, and bodies that are told two different truths by society and the medical establishment.

Because we do not have an adequate feminist discursive space from which to conceptualize the breastfeeding body, the human milk that has come to be so highly valued for its scientific properties remains rhetorically separate from the body of the mother who produces it. So even though we seem largely to agree that mothers should breastfeed for scientific reasons, we want nothing to do with the messy realities of the maternal and infant bodies that are neces-sarily involved in that activity. This situation creates some bizarre moments of tension in the public sphere. We have already discussed the periodic media reports about nursing mothers who are asked to leave restaurants or other public places even though they are not doing anything illegal or improper. But even more perplexing are situations in which people seem to feel uncom-fortable even looking at images of the breastfeeding body. For example, in Lubbock, Texas, in 2007, an artist was asked to remove from her exhibit a set of paintings that depicted mothers breastfeeding their babies.[5] Photos of breastfeeding mothers have even been removed from Facebook in recent years, presumably in response to user complaints about obscenity.[6] And when the Office of Women's Health spent forty million dollars on a breastfeeding promotion campaign, the advertising materials did not display actual women or babies engaged in the act of breastfeeding. Instead they displayed a variety of objects unrelated to breastfeeding or lactation (otoscopes, ice cream cones, and dandelion seed heads, to be exact) but positioned these objects in a way that vaguely resembled women's breasts.

It is useful now to reflect more explicitly on how some of the insights that emerge through understanding the kairology of infant feeding might help us expand feminist discursive spaces to account more fully for the embodied realities of breastfeeding, both past and present. In this discussion the term *feminist discursive space,* instead of *feminist discourse,* is often used to reflect the idea that, as we move forward with this effort, we need to interpret broadly the concept of discourse to mean a noisy banter—the kind of vibrant discussion in which feminist scholars will not fully agree, but in which the new ideas produced from the disagreement make the conversation worthwhile.

Feminism, Science, and Breastfeeding: Bringing the Problem into Clearer View

One of the most important themes that has emerged from our analysis is the way in which science has served as an ever-shifting frame for infant-feeding controversies in the United States. Specifically, mid-twentieth-century scientific research and clinical practice were framed by what we have identified as the topos of breastfeeding as foundation: the assumption that human milk was an ideal substance and, therefore, should be emulated in all attempts to produce and use artificial substitutes. By the end of the twentieth century, such research and clinical practice were coming to be defined by the dramatically different set of assumptions entailed in what we have called the topos of breastfeeding as the norm: the notion that human milk is the norm and, therefore, will never be adequately replaced by an artificial substitute. In the most recent times, as scientific evidence in support of breastfeeding has continued to accumulate, the topos of breastfeeding as the norm has started to develop into an emerging rhetorical framework that we have called the topos of formula as risky. Despite the changes and evolution that have occurred throughout this entire historical period, however, one aspect has remained constant: we have always required greater quantities and quality of scientific evidence to support positive claims about human milk than we have ever required of claims that are made about the safety or health-promoting qualities of formula.

These findings about the unevenness of the rhetorical situation faced by advocates of breastfeeding and bottle-feeding are important because they provide us with a more complete understanding of the situation that we currently face as scholars interested in expanding the feminist discursive space that surrounds breastfeeding. As we have seen, the kairology of U.S. infant-feeding policy and practice over the last several decades has been defined by an ever-intensifying and increasingly narrow focus on the scientific reasons for supporting breastfeeding. This narrow focus on science must be held at least partially responsible for our current tendency to ignore or exclude the breastfeeding body and to separate the embodied aspects of breastfeeding from the scientific properties of human milk that we now seem to understand so well. Bernice L. Hausman makes this argument in her most recent book, *Viral Mothers: Breastfeeding in the Age of HIV/AIDS*. Specifically, Hausman observes, the feminist debate that was sparked by the NBAC highlights the extent to which breastfeeding is narrowly circumscribed as a biomedical construct and how this situation precludes the possibility of making other kinds of arguments or statements about breastfeeding. As Hausman says, "These controversies, especially within feminist scholarship, demonstrate the difficulty of representing the value of women's bodies in anything other than medical terms."[7]

Adding some historical perspective to the situation that Hausman describes, our analysis has suggested that the new understanding of human milk's immune-protective qualities only became possible when human milk came to be seen as part of the gender-neutral immune system rather than primarily as a part of women's reproductive functions. In other words, we might say that scientific appreciation of human milk's health-promoting qualities has only been made possible by separating human milk from the maternal body that can produce and deliver it—the same separation, I would argue, that we see manifested on so many levels in popular culture today.

As feminist scholars interested in expanding the discursive space that supports breastfeeding, this means that we face an apparent dilemma. On the one hand, scientific arguments for human milk's health-promoting qualities have been the only successful way to restore medical appreciation for breastfeeding in the context of a long and persistent historical tendency to devalue this uniquely female capacity of the human body. As we have seen, when breastfeeding advocates in the late 1970s tried to accuse formula companies of unethical marketing practices, they did not succeed in convincing the AAP to adopt a stronger pro-breastfeeding stance; rather the AAP's 1982 policy statement essentially preserved the status quo at that time, which entailed a belief that formula and human milk were more or less equal. However, when breastfeeding advocates acquired evidence that was strong enough to support a scientific claim that human milk offers a unique form of immune protection that benefits infants even in developed countries, they were finally able to form a coalition and to persuade the AAP to declare breastfeeding the "reference or normative model" in their 1997 policy statement.

However, the exclusive focus on the science of breastfeeding, as we have suggested, is exacerbating the uncomfortable divide between human milk and all of the embodied aspects that surround lactation and breastfeeding for the mothers who continue to experience so many difficulties with regard to these aspects of life. An extraordinary amount of rhetorical effort has been required to reach a point where human milk is valued for the unique health benefits it is now seen to offer to the nursing infant and mother. Knowing this rhetorical history makes it all the more troubling that even now, after all of the rhetorical effort it has taken to get to the point where human milk has some scientific value, we have still not reached the point where our society values or even accepts the actual bodies of breastfeeding mothers. Clearly, even though we might have gained some appreciation of human milk as a scientific construct, we seem to want to pretend that breastfeeding itself does not exist, or at least that it does not matter to our society at large because it is something that the good mother will carry out behind the scenes, in her own home, at a time and place that will not inconvenience anyone else.

Any attempt to expand feminist discursive spaces must grapple with these competing demands to preserve the argumentative ground that has been gained through scientific arguments in favor of breastfeeding and, at the same time, to combat the persistent dissociation of breastfeeding from the maternal body that has occurred as a side effect of the narrow focus on scientific aspects of the breastfeeding relationship. The challenge, then, is to build and expand a discursive space that allows us to criticize some of the current trends in breast-feeding-promotion efforts but still sympathize with the larger goals of making breastfeeding more widely accepted as both a scientifically recommended form of infant nutrition *and* an embodied activity that sometimes gets in the way and disrupts our usual ways of doing things—not only for the mother and infant but for all of us as well. As feminist breastfeeding scholars, we cannot be satisfied with a world that continues to emphasize the scientific elements of breastfeeding at the expense of all other considerations.

Confronting New Challenges:
A Response to Joan B. Wolf

Because a rhetorical approach to infant feeding helps us more clearly define the historical dimensions of our present situation, I hope it might also prepare us to engage with the new challenges that will inevitably arise as we attempt to expand feminist discursive spaces for breastfeeding. Along these lines, it is especially important to respond to two recent texts that are posing new challenges for feminist scholars who support breastfeeding. Specifically, in a 2007 article, "Is Breast Really Best? Risk and Total Motherhood in the National Breastfeeding Awareness Campaign," and a 2011 book, *Is Breast Best? Taking on the Breastfeeding Experts and the New High Stakes of Motherhood,* Joan B. Wolf claims to offer the first pieces of scholarship that directly and boldly confront the "axiomatic" faith in breastfeeding that she sees as characterizing the medical community's current stance. Wolf's arguments center on two primary assertions. First, she contends that the scientific evidence invoked to support current breastfeeding promotion efforts such as the NBAC is weak because breastfeeding researchers have been too quick to equate correlation with causation. In Wolf's words, "an analysis of the epidemiological research on breastfeeding . . . indicates that while breastfed babies, on average, do appear to be slightly healthier, the science does not demonstrate compellingly that breast milk or breastfeeding is responsible."[8] Wolf's contention, repeated often throughout the book, is that there is no way to determine with certainty that it is the feeding method that is leading to the improved health outcomes for breastfed babies that tend to be reported in large clinical studies comparing breastfed and formula-fed babies. As she observes, it is possible that mothers who choose to breastfeed and are able to do so for the recommended length of time are also adopting other health-promoting behaviors, and, according to Wolf, the existing studies routinely cited to support messages that promote breastfeeding do not adequately control for these other factors. Wolf explains the tendency to distort the importance of scientific evidence on infant feeding in terms of a "total motherhood" ideology. Specifically, as she says, "total motherhood stipulates that mothers' primary occupation is to predict and prevent all less-than-optimal social, emotional, cognitive, and physical outcomes . . . and then any potential diminution in harm to children trumps all other considerations in risk analysis as long as mothers can achieve the reduction."[9] It is this tendency to emphasize the responsibilities as traditionally conceived in biological notions of motherhood, according to Wolf, that leads scientists, medical experts, and the public at large to place such a great emphasis on the importance of breastfeeding as a health-promoting behavior while ignoring other behaviors and decisions that could impact children's health.

The notion of a "total motherhood" ideology leads to Wolf's second main assertion, which is that the risk-based approach that the designers of the NBAC used to encourage breastfeeding was ethically inappropriate because it relies on and exploits popularly held distortions about risk in relation to infant feeding. Specifically, Wolf criticizes the NBAC because it "presented breastfeeding research as far more certain than it is and the risks of not breastfeeding as more severe than they would be even if the science were compelling."[10] Wolf argues that the campaign's risk-based approach was ethically problematic because "it capitalized on the public's general confusion about risk," and because "it embraced the principle that mothers have the unique capacity and obligation to protect their offspring from short- and long-term threats and that responsible mothers produce healthy babies."[11] In making the latter accusation, Wolf echoes concerns that other feminist scholars have expressed about the NBAC. However, whereas other feminist scholars have criticized the NBAC for its fear-based rhetorical tactics, Wolf goes one step further and questions the validity of the scientific evidence on which it was based.[12]

Wolf's ideas became controversial the moment they became available for public scrutiny. In fact, alongside Wolf's 2007 article, the *Journal of Health Politics, Policy and Law* published a commentary by Judy M. Hopkinson, lactation physiologist and faculty member in pediatrics at Baylor College of Medicine. Just a few months after Wolf's article appeared in print, the *Journal of Human Lactation* published a commentary by M. Jane Heinig, a well-respected board-certified lactation consultant. Both commentaries harshly refute Wolf's arguments with especially close scrutiny to her claims about breastfeeding science. However, such criticisms have not thwarted the popular uptake of Wolf's texts. As I write this chapter in early 2012, Wolf's 2007 article has already been cited forty-four times, according to GoogleScholar, and her 2011 book has been cited seven times. She has appeared on televised talk shows and as an invited speaker at numerous venues. By contrast, Hopkinson's commentary has been cited only six times, and Heinig's has been cited only four times. In other words, the published refutations of Wolf's arguments, both written by well-established experts in lactation science, have received far less public attention than Wolf's original arguments have received.

With the publication of Wolf's article and book, feminist scholars who are skeptical of the current medical enthusiasm for breastfeeding have gained some new ground. Although her book has not been available long enough to know exactly how it will shape future conversations, its immediate reception and public visibility indicate that it is likely to have some profound effects. But what about feminist scholars who are more inclined to support breastfeeding? How might we respond to Joan B. Wolf? In light of the high acclaim that her texts are receiving, how might feminist breastfeeding scholars productively engage with Wolf's arguments as we continue our efforts to expand the feminist discursive space for breastfeeding?

An important first step is to acknowledge the flaws that critics have pointed out in Wolf's scientific reasoning. As Hopkinson says at the beginning of her commentary, she chose to focus on Wolf's claims about the scientific evidence because that is the hardest part of Wolf's argument for a lay reader to evaluate. Specifically, Hopkinson states that her goals are to "focus on Joan Wolf's literature review" and to "direct the reader to other parts of Wolf's article requiring a critical eye."[13] Hopkinson asserts that Wolf lacks support for many of her statements. Hopkinson also strongly disagrees with Wolf's statement that gastrointestinal infections are not a serious problem in the United States. (Gastrointestinal infections are the one area in which Wolf concedes that the scientific evidence supports breastfeeding's benefits to the infant.) Hopkinson also says that scientific research on infant feeding is rapidly advancing and is undergoing some dramatic changes. In the near future, according to Hopkinson, we will have moved away from the simple question of breastfeeding versus formula-feeding. Instead, we will be able to look at specific components in human milk and to gain a better understanding of the various health benefits in their specificity.[14] Hopkinson takes issue with the manner in which Wolf interprets the findings of some of the studies that she reviews. For instance, in the research on ear infections that Wolf discusses, Hopkinson says that Wolf ignores some important studies. Hopkinson also accuses Wolf of glossing over one of the difficulties in infant-feeding research as it has usually been conducted: such research has not paid sufficient attention to the importance of exclusive breastfeeding.[15]

Heinig's commentary, published a few months after Wolf's 2007 article, also directly refutes Wolf's arguments and echoes Hopkinson's close scrutiny of Wolf's scientific claims and reasoning. In her refutation of Wolf's scientific arguments, Heinig acknowledges that infant-feeding research as a whole does not consistently support the health advantages of breastfeeding in industrialized countries and that there are some gaps and inconsistencies in this very large body of research. However, Heinig ascribes these gaps and inconsistencies to "the lack of consideration for duration and exclusivity of breastfeeding when classifying feeding groups." Furthermore, Heinig acknowledges these kinds of gaps and inconsistencies as a widespread problem in public health research: "Indeed, outcomes from studies of human health are rarely consistent."[16] Echoing Hopkinson's criticisms, Heinig also accuses Wolf of selectively reporting only the negative results from one institutional randomized clinical trial that is available. She also states that Wolf is wrong to claim that the mechanisms of breastfeeding's protection are poorly understood and provides a good amount of scientific detail to undermine Wolf's claims in this regard.

These two arguments against Wolf's interpretation of breastfeeding science are important to acknowledge. The careful reader will want to pay attention to the questions that these lactation experts pose in regard to Wolf's assessment of breastfeeding science. And from a rhetorical perspective, these critical commentaries are important reminders that, no matter how much Wolf's critique of breastfeeding science might be resonating with some readers, she is not likely to have the last word in this ongoing controversy. In fact, the argumentative trajectory that we have traced in this book might even offer a rhetorical explanation for the apparent success of the anti-breastfeeding arguments presented in Wolf's recent texts. Viewed in the context of this rhetorical history, we might understand the rhetorical success of Wolf's article and book as the latest in a long, ongoing series of rhetorical efforts to devalue human milk and breastfeeding by calling into question the motivations of those who make claims about their importance. Viewed from this perspective, Wolf's article and book are exposed as another stage in the persistent tendency to devalue breastfeeding and to place a much higher burden of proof on those who make claims in favor of breastfeeding than we have ever placed on claims about formula.

For these reasons, my own concerns about Wolf's texts, and particularly her book, echo the concerns that Hopkinson and Heinig express about Wolf's simplistic approach to current breastfeeding science. But I would like to expand on these two commentaries and express some additional concerns that arise from a rhetorical perspective on infant feeding. One concern about Wolf's book is the manner in which she characterizes the history of U.S. infant-feeding discourse. Her book devotes about one half of one chapter (twelve pages) to the history of infant-feeding practices in the United States from colonial times to the present.[17] She uses this history to situate the current pro-breastfeeding messages that are the primary focus of her book, and thus, in this twelve-page section, she emphasizes how each era has produced medical recommendations on infant feeding that have moved closer to today's total motherhood ideology in support of breastfeeding. To explain what she calls the "resurgence of breastfeeding" that has occurred since the 1960s, Wolf offers a brief explanation of the role that La Leche League played in mid-twentieth-century efforts to restore breastfeeding and then discusses efforts such as the Nestle Boycott and women's health movement that further consolidated interest in breastfeeding in the 1960s, 70s, and 80s.[18] Because this historical section attempts to cover the last several decades in only twelve pages, the analysis glosses over important moments of conflict that have preceded the present moment. It is because of this overly general characterization of infant-feeding history that Wolf is ultimately able to offer the one-dimensional notion of a total motherhood ideology as an explanation of the current resurgence of medical enthusiasm for breastfeeding. As our own rhetorical analysis has shown, there are many more factors at play in current discourses besides just biological notions about motherhood, and it is simplistic to equate the current pro-breastfeeding stance with anti-woman tendencies and to ignore the extent to which current discourses are responding to all of the anti-woman tendencies that preceded them. Wolf does identify several of the factors that converged to establish bottle-feeding as the norm after commercially produced formulas became available and became recognized as generally safe. However, she does not address the many nuances and points of conflict within medicine that have brought us to where we are today.

Of particular concern is the fact that so much medical discourse over the centuries, but especially in the twentieth century, has been devoted to comparing human milk unfavorably to its animal equivalents. And one of the major forces that caused such discourse to shift away from this negative stance toward the breastfeeding body, as we have seen, was a series of scientific discoveries that forced medicine to see breastfeeding as part of the immune system—a bodily system that is not connected to reproduction and, therefore, is seen as gender neutral rather than uniquely female. As I have suggested, it might not be just a coincidence that, after this shift occurred, breastfeeding suddenly gained more respect in the medical community and, consequently, the arguments of those experts who for many decades had been advocating breastfeeding suddenly made much more sense to medical audiences.

In ignoring the intricacies of this historical context, Wolf exacerbates the persistent tendency to isolate current breastfeeding discourse, seeming to put it on a stage all by itself without considering the long historical context of anti-breastfeeding sentiment that preceded today's pro-breastfeeding exhortations. As she observes, the amount of attention that researchers pay to breastfeeding continues to increase. It is hard to argue with that general observation. From a rhetorical perspective, though, we have to ask, would breastfeeding currently be receiving this much attention from researchers if there was not this persistent need to restore scientific faith in this aspect of women's bodies that has been so persistently denigrated for so long? If mid-twentieth-century researchers had not consistently perpetuated negative beliefs about this uniquely female bodily capacity, would we be in a position today that demands such a great deal of effort and attention to prove scientifically every possible health benefit that breastfeeding might offer to the mother and infant?

To ask these questions is of course not to deny that there could be anti-feminist tendencies in some of today's breastfeeding discourse. However, as I hope this book has made clear, such tendencies have to be understood in a context that is much more complicated than that which is acknowledged in a feminist critique such as Wolf's, which looks only at the current discourse without considering what that discourse is responding to. The current resurgence of medical enthusiasm for breastfeeding cannot be reduced to just a desire to put women back in the home and make them bound to exclusive mothering. Rather, as we have seen, today's enthusiastic pro-breastfeeding discourse is responding to a long history of battles against breastfeeding, and when we look at these battles, chart them as rhetorical struggles, their relationships to the ideologies of gender become much more murky and harder to define. Rather than dismiss the current breastfeeding fervor based on a surface reading of the highly visible discourses that we see in current public-health campaigns, this book has illuminated some of the historical reasons why these discourses are as fervent as they are.

For similar reasons, the analysis presented in chapter 2 also sheds new light on Wolf's suggestion that there is an anti-feminist bias in the current scientific research on the immune benefits of breastfeeding. A major criticism that Wolf repeatedly states is that scientific research on breastfeeding is biased or ideologically slanted to favor breastfeeding and that, as a result, many of today's public-health messages exaggerate the health benefits of breastfeeding. For instance, Wolf characterizes the medical support of breastfeeding as so widespread that the current research findings about human milk's immune protection are invalid—supporters are simply seeing what they want to see—and she even cites studies to support her claim that scientists routinely make this move. In Wolf's words: "To navigate this increasingly vast and labyrinthine terrain of research, scientists and physicians rely on conventional wisdom, and the more they do so, the more conventional the wisdom becomes. Trained in and habituated to risk-factor research and accustomed to news of breastfeeding's powers, they reproduce and have little reason to doubt positive findings."[19]

Wolf is correct to point out that many of today's studies begin with the assumption that breastfeeding will offer some form of immune protection. But her characterization of that tendency as a "bias" is questionable in light of the rhetorical history that we have reviewed. When we look at the history of scientific arguments about these immune-system benefits, we see that there has actually been a great deal of bias *against* such benefits. So if today's rhetoric seems passionate or overstated at times, that is probably because it is reacting against that long tradition. More specifically, as we have seen, immunologists have agreed since the 1970s that human milk contains a unique type of antibodies, and pediatricians have widely accepted this belief since at least the 1980s. The remaining questions have pertained to whether or not the immune protection afforded by human milk is necessary or significant in populations in the developed world today, where availability of antibiotics, a well-established health-care infrastructure, and relative cleanliness have made infant illnesses such as diarrhea and respiratory infections less of a direct threat to infant morbidity and mortality than they have been in the past (or still are in less developed countries). When we consider the full history of this ongoing debate, it might not be quite as surprising that many of today's studies would start with the assumption that human milk offers some form and level of immune-system protection, and just because the studies make this assumption explicit does not necessarily mean they do so because of the influence of a total motherhood ideology, as Wolf has said. Rather, their apparent bias might reflect the relatively certain scientific knowledge that human milk does contain immune-protective elements. Thus, it should be surprising to find out that protection *does not* seem to matter at statistically significant levels in some study populations, and it should not necessarily be so surprising when study results suggest that it *does* matter. Because the immune protection has long been clinically observed in some populations and has now also been well explained in the laboratory, the burden of proof should be placed on those who would demonstrate otherwise. But in the case of breastfeeding discourse, for the most part, that has not been true.

A second concern about Wolf's narrow focus on the present moment in current breastfeeding discourse is that it forecloses important questions that we might be asking about the present situation faced by breastfeeding mothers in the United States. For instance, in the case of examining the risk-based messages that were used in the NBAC advertising materials, one important consideration from a rhetorical perspective is that focus groups conducted before the advertising campaign suggested that scare tactics such as those used in the television ads would be the most effective way to persuade U.S. women that breastfeeding is worth their effort, in spite of all of the negative messages they had already heard from various sources about the experience of breastfeeding itself.[20] Rather than just condemning the ads themselves, as Wolf (and other feminist scholars) have done, I hope that the research presented in this book allows us to take the next step and ask what are the rhetorical forces that have transformed breastfeeding into an activity that is so dreaded and feared by large numbers of women that scare tactics have been deemed the most effective way to persuade them to do it? In fact, these focus-group participants' comments might be said to reflect the larger problem we have been describing: these participants seemed to value human milk as a scientific or nutritional substance but had many reservations about breastfeeding as an embodied activity in which they could successfully engage. Curiously, questions about these participant responses have not been asked in any of the public discourses surrounding the campaign or in the controversy that ultimately caused its messages to be watered down at the last minute.

Although Wolf is correct to point out that the current rhetorical formation is generating the strongest pro-breastfeeding messages that we have seen in recent times, it is also important to acknowledge the complexity of today's rhetorical situation. As in previous times, seemingly strong pro-breastfeeding messages from the public-health and medical establishments are being countered by messages from other sources. In fact, as the pro-breastfeeding messages have become increasingly strong, the rhetorical situation that frames arguments about both breast- and bottle-feeding seems to have become more polarized. Indeed, even though breastfeeding has become increasingly subject to medical attention in recent years, the discourses that shape the contours of this experience for any individual woman come from a variety of locations— not just from the physician who might inform her that exclusive breastfeeding is recommended for the first six months of an infant's life.

Numerous studies in public health have suggested how impactful these competing alternative discourses can be in shaping a mother's perceptions and experiences of infant feeding.[21] Many of these studies suggest that we still live in a culture in which messages that discourage breastfeeding far outweigh those that encourage it, even despite the strengthened medical support that breastfeeding appears to have received in recent years. This research also suggests that such discouraging messages prevent many mothers from breastfeeding altogether or cause them to wean earlier than they would otherwise desire. Findings such as these provide all the more reason why rhetoric should not be ignored if we hope to develop a complete picture of current beliefs and practices in regard to infant feeding. The real problem that we should all be fighting against is not that women are instructed to breastfeed, as Wolf says, but that they are told to do so in a world that, in every way imaginable, works against that possibility.

A third concern about Wolf's argument is her failure to offer any viable alternatives to the risk-based mentality of which she is so critical. As Wolf says, our collective eagerness to base our health-related decisions and practices on convincing scientific evidence and to alter those decisions and practices when the scientific wind shifts in a new direction is one of the characteristics that has made risk-based messages such as we see in the NBAC both effective and ethically suspect. Specifically, Wolf says we live in a "risk culture" and that this culture "structures how maternal responsibility is defined in public discourse, how breastfeeding advocates make claims about risk, and how the government uses fear to persuade women to breastfeed."[22] The concern about overreliance on scientifically calculated risks is an important one. However, I question whether Wolf's analysis really offers us a way out of this risk mentality. It seems that she just provides a different interpretation of the scientific evidence in hopes that it will lead us to a different decision: to bottle-feed instead of breastfeed. And given that most U.S. women still are not able to follow the recommendation to breastfeed exclusively for six months, it seems that Wolf's analysis might just reinforce these existing practices, even though she reinterprets the scientific evidence in a way that she hopes will make us all more accepting of the status quo. In other words, Wolf's analysis might serve to reinforce the very same risk-based mentality that she sets out to problematize. Furthermore, by singling out the scientific reasons for why women should make infant-feeding decisions, Wolf's text could be said to perpetuate the problematic divide between human milk as a scientific entity and the mother's body that can produce and deliver that milk.

This concern about Wolf's approach to risk-based thinking is probably the most pressing of the concerns mentioned because it requires us to move beyond the realm of scholarly debate to consider the practical implications of Wolf's texts for the many U.S. mothers who want to breastfeed but encounter obstacles at every step of the way. This is a point that Hopkinson expresses quite boldly in the commentary published along with Wolf's 2007 article. As

Hopkinson says, "Denying the value of breast-feeding in order to facilitate accommodation of inappropriate cultural pressures [as Wolf does] is neither an acceptable nor a responsible solution to our current dilemma. We can do better."[23] By exposing the multiple, conflicting discourses that continue to surround breastfeeding and influence mothers' decision-making processes, I hope that this book's rhetorical analysis has suggested some specific ways in which we might, as Hopkinson says, "do better" for the many women who really want to breastfeed and are made unable for reasons that have nothing to do with researchers studying the scientific aspects of human milk and breastfeeding in individuals and populations.

Finally, although this concern about Wolf's failure to offer an alternative to the risk-based mentality that she criticizes is the most pressing of the three concerns discussed, it is also the aspect of Wolf's arguments that presents the greatest opportunities for feminist scholars interested in expanding the discursive space for breastfeeding in the United States. In articulating a feminist response to Wolf, it is important to move beyond the quibbles over scientific evidence that have been such a prominent defining feature of infant-feeding controversies throughout the historical period that we have examined. In fact, as feminist breastfeeding scholars, we might even see Wolf's texts as an invitation to expand the types of arguments that we are able to make in support of breastfeeding. I hope that continued efforts to understand the kairology of infant feeding might open our eyes to an alternative to the risk-based mentality that Wolf correctly identifies as so pervasive in our culture.

I would even like to hope that we could get to a place where infant feeding and other health-related decisions would be understood in ways that escape the risk-mentality and cost-benefits kind of thinking of which Wolf is so deeply critical. I have argued that strong scientific arguments have been a necessary component of breastfeeding advocates' efforts to restore medical faith in breastfeeding. But maybe we could eventually get beyond these scientific arguments and arrive at pro-breastfeeding arguments that consider more than just science, and maybe Wolf's efforts to debunk breastfeeding science are the exigency that will force us to make that next move. Maybe an expanded feminist discursive space would provide room for mothers to express a desire to breastfeed, and even to claim it as a right, for reasons that are other than scientific. All of these things are included in what might be called the embodied rhetoric of mothering—a potentially powerful rejoinder to the popular images of disembodied motherhood presented at the beginning of this chapter. Maybe there are reasons to breastfeed that extend beyond the scientifically informed, risk-aware "good mother" mentality that Wolf provides as the only explanation for why a woman would want to breastfeed, and maybe, as we continue to expand the feminist discursive space for breastfeeding, we will open up new possibilities for building effective arguments in this regard.

Expanding beyond the scientific arguments that have been so successful in supporting breastfeeding mothers is a potentially risky argumentative strategy because it might require us to accept that the science will never be certain, that there will always be new questions, and that breastfeeding will always, to some extent, be put on the defensive in situations where it is held up for comparison against formula-feeding. We must remember, though, that there is also a risk involved in remaining so closely focused on the scientific debate that we neglect other aspects of breastfeeding, human milk, and lactation. We cannot forget, for instance, that even if current medical consensus appears "axiomatic," as Wolf says, the biggest problem that today's mothers face is all of the conflicting messages that interfere with breastfeeding even for those mothers who really want to do it and should be able to. Mothers in these situations do not need more scientific evidence to demonstrate that breastfeeding promotes infant and maternal health; they need a world that is more supportive in every way of their efforts to breastfeed, for whatever reason they might offer for wanting to do that.

In short, as we expand feminist discursive spaces for breastfeeding, we need to resist the persistent tendency to separate human milk as a scientific substance from the embodied act and reality of the maternal breastfeeding body. It is that persistent separation, I would argue, that allows a text such as Wolf's *Is Breast Best?* to explain today's pro-breastfeeding discourse in terms of total motherhood. If we lived in a society that more fully valued breastfeeding itself, not just human milk as a scientific element, Wolf's arguments would not have the persuasive force that they currently have.

Closing Thoughts

Clearly the rhetorical contest that we have come to know as "breast or bottle" is far from over. Although there has been a dramatic shift in the contours of this rhetorical contest, the ground is still settling, and it would be incorrect to conclude that breastfeeding has won out forever or that the contest is over. Even as medically sanctioned pro-breastfeeding messages seem to be becoming more strident and more highly visible, the demands for more and better scientific evidence to support these messages continue to increase. As we have seen, formula companies have continued to find new ways to promote their products and have even been able to co-opt the ideas from current breastfeeding discourse, such as claims about immune protection, that have been most effective in asserting human milk's uniqueness and superiority over artificial substitutes. Women also continue to receive conflicting messages from less formal sources such as friends, relatives, and the culture at large, and these conflicting messages continue to make breastfeeding difficult even as official medical discourse claims to support it.

The deep rhetorical contradictions that have emerged indicate how far the notion of "normal" breastfeeding has come at the level of officially sanctioned discourse, but also how far is our culture at large from accepting breastfeeding as a normal activity. Although official discourses such as those produced by the AAP and circulated through the air waves by the NBAC have declared breastfeeding the norm, or even the only safe option, and although these authoritative sources have encouraged its acceptance from the top down, there is much available evidence to suggest that this is not an accurate description of breastfeeding as an actual embodied practice for many women who attempt it in the United States today.

Now, perhaps more than ever before, rhetorical analysis can provide the knowledge about infant feeding, past and present, that can empower parents to confront these conflicting discourses and thus engage more effectively in a "rhetorical care of the self" with regard to their infant-feeding decisions and experiences.[24] Thinking in these terms might provide a powerful antidote to the notion of individual choice that is so pervasive with regard to a wide array of women's health issues, but is at the same time so inadequate. I hope that it also might contribute to ongoing efforts to develop a feminist discourse of breastfeeding by providing powerful reminders of the embodied aspects of lactation and mothering that are so persistently ignored and excluded from today's public discourse on all sides of the breastfeeding controversy.

As we have seen, the maternal body is perhaps now more than ever besieged by rhetoric on all sides of the infant-feeding question—not just from the medical establishment but from all stakeholders. Although his words date back to the fourth century B.C.E., Gorgias' message about the unique form of power that rhetoric wields in the domain of health and medicine remains true: the skilled rhetor can often succeed at getting the patient to follow doctor's orders when the doctor fails. And this is a message that would not be lost on today's producers of infant-feeding messages on either side of the ongoing breast–bottle controversy. For every dollar that breastfeeding advocacy organizations spend on educating mothers about the health benefits and practical aspects of breastfeeding, formula companies spend many more dollars sending free samples to the homes of new and expecting mothers, sponsoring educational events for physicians, and purchasing expensive print, radio, Internet, and television advertisements.[25]

By drawing critical attention to all of these conflicting discourses, I hope this book contributes to current efforts to expand the feminist discursive space for breastfeeding and that it offers a decidedly different stance from those which are currently being brought to the table by parties on either side of this increasingly polarized conversation. I believe many of the current feminist efforts are misguided in taking such an adamant stance against one particular vein of pro-breastfeeding discourse—that of public-health efforts. There is much more going on here, both within medicine and in the larger culture. What we should be arguing against is the paralyzing situation that pits medical advice against the lived realities of motherhood and thus makes it virtually impossible for many women to adhere to the pro-breastfeeding recommendations that seem to be supported so strongly by the public face of today's medical establishment. As we have seen, today's enthusiastic medical support of breastfeeding is the product of a decades-long battle, which has been quite intense at times, to bring medical practice in line with scientific evidence. Although cultural constructions of motherhood have certainly been at stake in this rhetorical struggle, they have not been the critical turning point in the recent shift in medical stance toward breastfeeding. To argue strictly against the surface appearance of these medical recommendations and to ignore the larger context in which they occur is reductive, and it is a waste of energy. Whether we agree with all of the current medical recommendations or not, I would hope we could all agree that all women should live in a world where it is possible for mothers who so desire to adopt the behaviors that medicine currently recommends as most supportive of mothers' and infants' health.

Of course, the findings presented in this book are based on qualitative research, and as such they cannot be generalized to the entire U.S. population, nor can I claim that they represent U.S. breastfeeding discourse in its entirety. However, consistent with the book's grounding in rhetoric, which has a long tradition of emphasizing the particular as well as the general, this book has aimed to draw attention to the complexities that can exist in a particular moment, even if those particulars cannot be generalized to larger populations or deemed absolutely true in all times and places. Yes, there other epistemological frameworks that we can use to understand human communication—some far more systematic and thus better equipped for producing messages whose effectiveness we can predict with more scientific certainty. Studies in public health, for instance, have made great strides in tracking U.S. breastfeeding rates and how these rates break down across demographic lines. These studies have also usefully illuminated the obstacles to breastfeeding that exist for women in various demographic groups and allowed us to draw generalized conclusions about the best ways to design messages for these groups. But this book is grounded on the premise that sometimes, in addition to forming new generalizations, it is important to slow down and look at things in their particularity—in Aristotle's words, to examine the "given case" for what it is worth, rather than treating it simply as a representative example of something larger. In the wake of movements such as evidence-based medicine, it is easy to overlook the power of particulars. Thus, it is easy to forget that even amid the generalizations, there are exceptions, and these exceptions deserve to be studied for what they are worth in their own right, not just as part of a larger whole.

In more concrete terms, when we consider how wrong it is for the breast-feeding relationship to be unnecessarily disrupted by members of the same medical establishment who encourage women to do it, it is clear that even if that happens one time, it is worthy of notice and deserving of scholarly attention. As the data in this book have revealed, chapter 5 in particular, this type of situation has clearly been encountered by more than one breastfeeding woman in the last several years, which is all the more reason to devote our attention to it.

Toward this goal of understanding some of the particular situations that constitute the larger phenomenon of "breast or bottle" as we know it today, it has been my goal to take a multimodal, interdisciplinary approach to breastfeeding studies. Although rhetorical analysis is at the heart of my approach, I have attempted to expand on traditional techniques and principles of rhetorical analysis in some important ways. For example, I have not limited my approach to the strictly text-based analysis that we often see in traditional rhetoric-of-science studies. Rather, mine could be called a "rhetoric of the streets," or what Carl Herndl calls "critical practice."[26] My starting place has been scientific and medical texts, but I have tried not to look at these texts as something produced only for other scientific and medical experts; rather, I have looked at some of the ways in which these texts frame the lived experience of breastfeeding for actual women, and I have done so by listening to the words of women themselves who have experienced breastfeeding from many different social and geographic locations. At the same time, I have also incorporated data from interviews with breastfeeding experts, people who have been involved in producing the expert discourses to which today's mothers are repeatedly exposed. Some previous analyses have used these approaches, but most have chosen one or the other: either strictly textual analysis or strictly interview-based research. For instance, there is an emerging feminist interest in critiquing the scientific and medical discourses.[27] However, these analyses so far have been strictly text-based, not incorporating interviews or other field research. There is also a growing body of literature, especially in public health and the social sciences, that tries to understand women's breastfeeding experiences on their own terms. However—maybe with the exception of Linda M. Blum's *At the Breast*—this research tends to take the scientific and medical discourses for granted; it does not question the scientific validity of "breast is best" but instead uses qualitative research as a way to try to understand why so many women fail to breastfeed despite this scientific knowledge.

In taking an interdisciplinary, multimodal approach, I have tried to combine what is best from the textual analysis studies and the ethnographic studies, from the humanities and the social sciences, providing a picture of current U.S. breastfeeding practices that is unique in its interdisciplinary orientation and its multifaceted methodological approach. Truly to articulate a feminist discourse on breastfeeding, we need to hear from women themselves, along with the various scientific, medical, and popular texts on which other feminist scholars, such as Jules Law and Bernice L. Hausman, have based their arguments for a feminist discourse. So my method is rhetorical analysis, but it does not isolate the scientific and medical texts from their contexts and audiences in the way that traditional approaches to textual analysis have sometimes done.

Rather than continuing to criticize the pro-breastfeeding messages in their own right, and viewing such discourses in a vacuum, apart from historical context, a rhetorical analysis foregrounds the continuing proliferation and viral nature of conflicting discourses about infant feeding as the root of mothers' confusion about and resistance to the expert discourses of infant feeding. A rhetorical approach to infant feeding also leads us to question the illusion of choice as it exists in the context of conflicting messages that circulate about a subject such as infant feeding: a phrase such as *breast or bottle* conceals the manner in which multiple discourses of infant feeding compete for dominion over a mother's choice by exploiting or dismissing the "scientific." The choice between breast and bottle is not a reality but a powerful rhetorical fabrication.

As much as this book is an argument for a particular approach to a feminist discourse on breastfeeding, it is also an argument for truly interdisciplinary research and multimodal approaches to health-related topics such as infant feeding. Although breastfeeding has dimensions that are scientific, dimensions that are medical, and dimensions that are cultural, any woman who has ever attempted breastfeeding in recent U.S. history knows that in the actual embodied experience, these dimensions cannot be neatly separated from one another. My study starts from this perspective. In striving for a truly interdisciplinary approach, I strive to achieve what Ellen Barton has called "disciplined interdisciplinarity"—that is, research with elements that can be understood by audiences in more than one discipline.[28] In so doing, I have been a critically engaged researcher, studying breastfeeding in all of its various dimensions, not only as a scholarly researcher but also as a breastfeeding mother and activist.

One of the most important insights that strikes me as I reflect on the many hours of research and writing that have culminated in this book is the extent to which breastfeeding in our culture is persistently and intentionally claimed as a political cause by so many different segments of society. The medical community touts it as the key to lifelong health for mother and baby, La Leche League depicts it as the key to perfect parenting, and public-health initiatives promote it as a quick fix to a variety of social ills. However, at the same time websites and books are passionately devoted to reassuring bottle-feeding mothers that they should not feel guilty for their decision to abandon breastfeeding or never even try it in the first place.[29]

On a more personal level, I began to experience the ideologically charged nature of infant feeding when my first child was born, about thirteen years ago. Throughout my pregnancy, I was bombarded with propaganda from both sides—the formula companies sent me gallons of free formula in the mail while my health-care providers made sure I knew the benefits of breastfeeding and encouraged me to sign up for a prenatal breastfeeding class. Once the baby was born, the pressure from all sides became even more intense. Almost immediately after my child's birth, lactation consultants were by my side and willing to stay there as long as necessary until a suitable latch-on was achieved, but in the wee hours of my son's fussy, exhausting second night of life, a labor and delivery nurse suggested I feed him a bottle of formula to help him sleep. In my first few weeks at home, I successfully established breastfeeding, but it seemed as if the baby would never want to do anything else. When well-meaning relatives and friends called from all over the country to ask how I was doing, and I said I was exhausted from feeding the baby so much, more than one urged me to try just an occasional bottle of formula to fill his belly and help him sleep more soundly.

Now that my oldest son is thirteen years old and has been joined by two younger siblings, I am still frequently reminded of the ideologically infused dimensions of the infant-feeding experience. In fact, with both of the younger children, I have had just as many anti-breastfeeding encounters with individuals in the health-care establishment and larger community as I did with the first one. Most recently, when my youngest son was about eight months old, a family physician told me I would need to wean him immediately if she referred me for a chest X-ray to diagnose pneumonia. (To this day, I am still not sure whether she was worried about the milk causing problems for the X-ray or the X-ray causing problems in the milk). Thankfully, I am well informed enough to know better (and I had health insurance that allowed me to switch to a different physician right away). Sadly, for many patients in that position, this incorrect, misguided advice would have caused them to wean right away.

One of the ways I believe that these types of difficult situations persist is through rhetorical isolation of this part of life from other aspects of women's health and the daily realities of women's lives. As has been suggested in this book, the attempt to establish breastfeeding as a normative model does represent a genuine effort on the part of the medical community to respond to women's demands for more and better medical information about breastfeeding. However, we have also seen that the normalizing stance being adopted reflects medicine's ever-present desire to reduce aspects of life such as infant feeding to purely clinical or scientific problems that can be addressed through overly simplified messages advising mothers that "breast is best" and that they can guarantee a positive breastfeeding experience by simply avoiding supplements in the early days of feeding so that their bodies will establish a healthy milk supply. By focusing on the scientific reasons why women should breastfeed their babies and downplaying or oversimplifying the social and political factors that contribute to any individual mother's decision to breastfeed or not, and her chances of being capable of continuing to breastfeed, today's medical discourse on breastfeeding is able to present itself outwardly as responding to women's demands while at the same time carefully maintaining its authority over this aspect of women's reproductive lives.

My ultimate aim in this book, then, has not been to argue either for or against breastfeeding but to answer Hausman's call for a feminist discourse on breastfeeding and to argue that such discourse is necessarily multiple and conflicting. On the one hand, feminist scholars need actively to critique the prevailing scientific and medical discourses on breastfeeding, but, on the other, they need to work against the tendency for these discourses to become isolated from the cultural realities of breastfeeding as an embodied experience or activity. One of the first steps is to unpack the myth that the science and medicine of breastfeeding are one and the same. If breastfeeding scholars focus exclusively on such discourses, we perpetuate the tendency to isolate scientific and medical discourse from other ways of understanding breastfeeding. We not only obscure the cultural dimensions but also preclude possibilities for finding ways to understand breastfeeding as a truly multifaceted phenomenon. Maybe it is possible to create new discursive spaces for knowing and talking about this aspect of life in ways that are neither scientific nor cultural, but somewhere between, and containing elements of both. Breastfeeding is, after all, not just an option that some mothers choose; it is also an embodied practice that, for a relatively short time in the span of raising a child, alters how we think about the maternal body in relation to the infant and thus demands a new way of thinking about nursing mothers' and infants' bodies and the boundaries between them.

Appendix

Research Participants

Key { *Pseudonym • Date of participation • Place of participation*
Participant description at time of participation

Alexia • July 31, 2008 • Lubbock, Tex.

Alexia participated in a focus group conducted at a community organization that provides prenatal support and education for underprivileged and single mothers in the Lubbock, Tex., area. She indicated her age as 18–24 years old, her occupation as unemployed, and her racial identity as African American. She had two children: a 19-month-old and a one-month-old. She described the feeding method for both children as mixed (both breast and bottle, and including solid foods for the older one).

Andrea • September 17, 2008 • Lubbock, Tex.

Andrea participated in a focus group conducted in 2008 at Texas Tech University. She indicated her age as 35–39 years old, her occupation as professional/administrative, and her racial identity as white. She had breastfed her first child until the age of six months and her second child until the age of five months.

Angelica • September 30, 2008 • Lubbock, Tex.

Angelica participated in a focus group conducted at Texas Tech University. She indicated her age as 25–29 years old, her occupation as unemployed, and her racial identity as white. She had a two-year-old child who had been breastfed exclusively until the age of five months, and she was expecting her second child.

Appendix

Carrie • July 4, 2005 • Lubbock, Tex.

Carrie participated in an individual interview. She was not employed outside the home. Her racial identity was white. She had one daughter who was four years old. She had breastfed her daughter for only a few days and then switched to the bottle. She fed the baby pumped breast milk for about a month and then switched to formula.

Connie • November 18, 2008 • Lubbock, Tex.

Connie participated in a focus group conducted at a community organization that provides prenatal support and education for underprivileged and single mothers in the Lubbock, Tex., area. She indicated her age as 18–24 years old, her occupation as health care/nonphysician, and her racial identity as white. She was expecting her first child.

Danielle • September 17, 2008 • Lubbock, Tex.

Danielle participated in a focus group conducted at Texas Tech University. She indicated her age as 18–24 years old, her occupation as retail, and her racial identity as white. She had a ten-month-old daughter, and she had breastfed for a short time when the baby was a newborn but then switched to formula.

Diane • April 24, 2000 • Minneapolis, Minn.

Diane participated in an individual interview. She had been working as a postpartum doula for seven years. Her racial identity was white. She had breastfed both of her children, each for at least one year.

Ellen • July 5, 2000 • Minneapolis, Minn.

Ellen participated in an individual interview. She had been working as a La Leche League leader for one year. Her racial identity was white. Ellen had breastfed one child until the age of 15 months. She was nursing her second child who was still an infant.

Grace • July 15, 2005 • Lubbock, Tex.

Grace participated in an individual interview. Her racial identity was white. She was employed as a personal trainer and sports nutritionist. She had two children, ages 11 and 9. She had breastfed both children for at least one year.

Jackie • July 11, 2000 • Minneapolis, Minn.

Jackie participated in an individual interview. She had been a La Leche League leader for ten years. Her racial identity was white. She had breastfed all three of her children, each for at least one year.

Janet • April 19, 2000 • Minneapolis, Minn.

Janet participated in an individual interview. She had been a La Leche League leader for 20 years and a board-certified lactation consultant for 15 years. Her racial identity was white. She had breastfed both of her children, each for at least one year.

Jessica • July 7, 2008 • Lubbock, Tex.

Jessica participated in a focus group conducted at Texas Tech University. She indicated her age as 18–24 years old, her occupation as unemployed, and her racial identity as Hispanic/Latino. She had an eight-month-old daughter, and she described her feeding methods as mixed (breast milk, formula, and some solid foods).

Jill • July 31, 2008 • Lubbock, Tex.

Jill participated in a focus group conducted at a community organization that provides prenatal support and education for underprivileged and single mothers in the Lubbock, Tex., area. She indicated her age as 18–24 years old, her occupation as office/clerical, and her racial identity as white. She had one child, and she described her feeding methods as mixed (both breast milk and formula).

Julie • July 31, 2008 • Lubbock, Tex.

Julie participated in a focus group conducted at a community organization that provides prenatal support and education for underprivileged and single mothers in the Lubbock, Tex., area. She indicated her age as 18–24 years old, her occupation as unemployed, and her racial identity as white. She had a two-week-old daughter, and she described her feeding methods as mixed (both breast milk and formula).

Karen • June 2, 2000 • Minneapolis, Minn.

Karen participated in an individual interview. She had been working as a board-certified lactation consultant for 19 years. Her racial identity was white. She had breastfed all four of her children for at least one year.

Kim • June 13, 2000 • Minneapolis, Minn.

Kim participated in an individual interview. She had been working as a La Leche League leader for three years. Her racial identity was white. She had breastfed all three of her children for at least one year.

Lisa • May 22, 2000 • Minneapolis, Minn.

Lisa participated in an individual interview. She had been a La Leche League leader for ten years. Her racial identity was white. She had breastfed her daughter for at least one year.

Mark • August 5, 2008 • Lubbock, Tex.

Mark participated in a focus group conducted at a community organization that provides prenatal support and education for underprivileged and single mothers in the Lubbock, Tex., area. He was attending the focus group with his spouse, Maria, who was expecting her first child. She indicated her age as 25–29 years old, her occupation as student, and her racial identity as white.

Mary • September 16, 2008 • Lubbock, Tex.

Mary participated in a focus group conducted in 2008 at Texas Tech University. She indicated her age as 30–34 years old, her occupation as unemployed, and her racial identity as white. She had two young children and had exclusively breastfed both children until the age of six months.

Michelle • June 1, 2000 • Minneapolis, Minn.

Michelle participated in an individual interview. She had been a La Leche League leader for about two years. Her racial identity was white. She had three children, including a set of twins. She had nursed all of her children for at least one year.

Nancy • September 24, 2008 • Lubbock, Tex.

Nancy participated in a focus group conducted in 2008 at Texas Tech University. She indicated her age as 25–29 years old, her occupation as unemployed, and her racial identity as white. She had exclusively breastfed her child until the age of five months.

Rebecca • August 5, 2008 • Lubbock, Tex.

Rebecca participated in a focus group conducted in 2008 at a community organization that provides prenatal support and education for underprivileged and single mothers in the Lubbock, Tex., area. She indicated her age as 18–24 years old, her occupation as restaurant/food service, and her racial identity as white. She was expecting her first child.

Sharon • March 31, 2000 • Minneapolis, Minn.

Sharon participated in an individual interview. She had been working as a board-certified lactation consultant for three years. Her racial identity was white. She had breastfed both of her children for at least one year.

Theresa • August 5, 2008 • Lubbock, Tex.

Theresa participated in a focus group conducted at a community organization that provides prenatal support and education for underprivileged and single mothers in the Lubbock, Tex., area. She indicated her age as 18–24 years old, her occupation as unemployed, and her racial identity as white. She was expecting her first child.

Tracy • July 31, 2008 • Lubbock, Tex.

Rebecca participated in a focus group conducted at a community organization that provides prenatal support and education for underprivileged and single mothers in the Lubbock, Tex., area. She indicated her age as 18–24 years old, her occupation as unemployed, and her racial identity as mixed race. She had two children: a four-year-old and a five-month-old. She had breastfed the oldest until he was eight weeks old, and she had formula-fed the youngest from birth.

Trisha • April 5, 2005 • Lubbock, Tex.

Trisha participated in an individual interview. She had been working as a labor doula and childbirth educator for about three years. She indicated her racial identity as white. She had three children, and all had been breastfed for at least one year. She was still nursing the youngest, who was about 18 months old at the time of the interview.

Notes

Introduction

1. Tomasi, introduction, xiii.

2. American Academy of Family Physicians Breastfeeding Advisory Committee, "Breastfeeding, Family Physicians Supporting (Position Paper)," para. 8.

3. AAP Work Group on Breastfeeding, "Breastfeeding and the Use of Human Milk," 496.

4. Aristotle, *Rhetoric*, 35.

5. Britt, *Conceiving Normalcy*; Segal, *Health and the Rhetoric of Medicine*; Emmons, *Black Dogs and Blue Words*.

6. "Babies Were Born to be Breastfed," U.S. Department of Health and Human Services, http://www.womenshealth.gov/breastfeeding/government-in-action/national -breastfeeding-campaign/adcouncil/babies.pdf (accessed May 8, 2012); "Breastmilk: Every Ounce Counts," Texas WIC Program, http://www.breastmilkcounts.com/ (accessed May 8, 2012).

7. Segal, *Health and the Rhetoric of Medicine*, 22.

8. Ibid., 23.

9. "'Log Rolling' Spot Transcript," National Women's Health Information Center, http://www.womenshealth.gov/breastfeeding/government-in-action/national-breast feeding-campaign/adcouncil/transcript_logroll.txt (accessed May 8, 2012).

10. Wolf, *Is Breast Best?* For a similar argument against the scientific evidence in support of breastfeeding, see also Law, "Politics of Breastfeeding," 412.

11. Kukla, "Ethics and Ideology," 159.

12. For similar arguments, see Friedman, "For Whom Is Breast Best?," and Knaak, "Deconstructing Discourse."

13. Hausman, *Mother's Milk*, 197–98.

14. Ibid., 15.

15. Friedman, "For Whom Is Breast Best?"; Knaak, "Deconstructing Discourse"; Kukla, "Ethics and Ideology"; Law, "Politics of Breastfeeding"; Wolf, *Is Breast Best?*

16. For more complete discussion and analysis of the medicalization of infant feeding, see Apple, *Mothers and Medicine*; Apple, *Perfect Motherhood*; Blum, *At the Breast*; Kukla, *Mass Hysteria*.

17. Emmons, *Black Dogs and Blue Words*, 7.

18. Relevant studies in public health include Cricco-Lizza, "Infant-Feeding Beliefs" and "Milk of Human Kindness"; Guttman and Zimmerman, "Low-Income Mothers' Views"; Khoury et al., "Breast-Feeding Initiation"; Mozingo et al., "'It Wasn't Working.'"

19. Segal, *Health and the Rhetoric of Medicine*, 2.

20. Selzer, "Rhetorical Analysis," 281.

21. Several recent books examine contemporary breastfeeding discourse without exploring its historical roots in much depth. See, for example, Bartlett, *Breastwork;* Blum, *At the Breast;* Carter, *Feminism, Breasts, and Breast-Feeding.;* Hausman, *Mother's Milk;* and Wolf, *Is Breast Best?* However, breastfeeding, and infant feeding more generally, have also received a great deal of attention from medical historians who each focus on a particular historical era. See, for example, Apple, *Mothers and Medicine;* Golden, *Social History of Wet Nursing;* Wolf, *Don't Kill Your Baby;* Yalom, *History of the Breast.* My approach differs from both of these categories of previous infant-feeding scholarship in that I analyze texts and events from both the past and the present. This approach is similar to that of other recent studies of medical rhetoric, including Berkenkotter, *Patient Tales;* Emmons, *Black Dogs and Blue Words;* Popham, "Forms as Boundary Genres"; Reeves, "Establishing a Phenomenon" and "Language, Rhetoric, and AIDS"; and Teston, "Grounded Investigation of Genred Guidelines."

22. Throughout the book, I use pseudonyms to protect interviewees' identities. The one exception is Dr. Lawrence Gartner, whom I interviewed by telephone on two different occasions. Quotations from these two interviews are included in a few places throughout the book and are clearly identified as such. All phases of the interview and focus-group research were approved by the Institutional Review Board at one or more research institutions.

23. Creswell, *Qualitative Inquiry,* 125.

24. Ibid., 128.

Chapter 1: Infant Feeding and Rhetoric

1. AAP Work Group on Breastfeeding, "Breastfeeding and the Use of Human Milk," 1035.

2. Ibid.

3. Ibid.

4. AAP Section on Breastfeeding, "Breastfeeding and the Use of Human Milk," 496.

5. See McCarthy and Gerring, "Revising Psychiatry's Charter Document," for a similar argument about medical discourse and narrative progress. McCarthy and Gerring make similar observations about the language used to justify changes in psychiatry's diagnostic categories. Specifically, McCarthy and Gerring identify two rhetorical strategies that authors used to justify the revisions they were recommending to the older version of psychiatry's diagnostic manual. On the one hand, the "Contingent Repertoire Account" was used to assure readers that the new version of the document would be more scientific than the older version, because it would not be influenced by "contingent or nonscientific factors, like personal and professional biases" (164). On the other hand, the "Progress of Science Account" was used to "emphasize the inevitability, the impersonality of the advance of the DSM" (167).

6. See the appendix for more detailed information on each of the research participants who are quoted in this chapter. The names that I use are pseudonyms. In the appendix the details about each participant are arranged in alphabetical order by pseudonym.

7. Fahnestock, "Accommodating Science," 279.

8. Segal, *Health and the Rhetoric of Medicine,* 23.

9. Mol, *Body Multiple,* viii; Leach and Dysart-Gale, "Why Ask Rhetorical Questions?," 1. See also Clarke et al., "Biomedicalization"; Löwy, *Between Bench and Bedside;* Mykhalovskiy, McCoy, and Bresalier, "Compliance/Adherence."

10. Miller, "Aristotelian *Topos*," 132.

11. Apple, *Mothers and Medicine*; Apple, *Perfect Motherhood*; Wolf, *Don't Kill Your Baby*.

12. Apple, *Mothers and Medicine*, 47–49.

13. Ibid., 72–73.

14. Apple, *Mothers and Medicine*; Apple, *Perfect Motherhood*; Baumslag and Michels, *Milk, Money, and Madness*; Blum, *At the Breast*.

15. Apple, *Mothers and Medicine*, 84–85; Apple, *Perfect Motherhood*; Blum, *At the Breast*, 30.

16. Sawicki, *Disciplining Foucault*, 76; Wolf, *Don't Kill Your Baby*, 160; Wolf, "What Feminists Can Do."

17. Apple, *Mothers and Medicine*, 35–49.

18. Cited in Apple, *Mothers and Medicine*, 56; also cited in Blum, *At the Breast*, 30.

19. Apple, *Mothers and Medicine*, 35–37.

20. Ibid., 73.

21. Scott, *Risky Rhetoric*, 61.

22. Clifford et al., "Panel Discussion," 108.

23. Ibid., 109.

24. Powers, "Some Observations on Feeding Premature Infants," 145, 155.

25. Dancis, Osborn, and Julia, "Studies of the Immunology of the Newborn Infant," 395.

26. Ibid.

27. Ward, *La Leche League*, 14.

28. AAP Work Group on Breastfeeding, "Breastfeeding and the Use of Human Milk," 1035.

29. AAP Task Force on the Promotion of Breast Feeding, "Promotion of Breastfeeding."

30. Ibid., 658, 660.

31. AAP Work Group on Breastfeeding, "Minutes," February 12, 1995.

32. AAP Work Group on Breastfeeding, "Breastfeeding and the Use of Human Milk," 1035.

33. For instance, breastfeeding receives some attention in the chapter entitled "Post Partum" in the course materials that were eventually published as the first edition of *Our Bodies, Ourselves*. Boston Women's Health Collective, *Women and Their Bodies: A Course* (Boston: Boston Women's Health Collective, 1970), accessed May 12, 2011, from http://www.ourbodiesourselves.org/uploads/pdf/OBOS1970.pdf.

34. "About ABM," Academy of Breastfeeding Medicine, http://www.bfmed.org/About/Default.aspx (accessed May 9, 2012).

35. AAP Section on Breastfeeding, "Breastfeeding and the Use of Human Milk," 497.

36. For a comprehensive review of current medical literature on the immunology of human milk, see Lawrence and Pane, "Human Breast Milk"; Lawrence and Pane's review is useful not only because of its thoroughness, but also because it suggests how the current "battle lines" are drawn between those who advocate human milk for its uniquely available immune-protective properties and those who emphasize the uncertainty in current scientific knowledge about those properties.

37. "HHS Blueprint for Action on Breastfeeding," U.S. Department of Health and Human Services, http://www.womenshealth.gov/breastfeeding/government-programs/hhs-blueprints-and-policy-statements/index.cfm#a (accessed May 8, 2012).

38. McKinney & Silver LLC, "National Breastfeeding Campaign."

39. Ibid., 204.

40. Ibid., 207.

41. The images of the insulin syringe and the asthma inhaler are available at http://img.photobucket.com/albums/v102/mysticirishwolf/breastfeeding%20campaign/nippleinsulin.gifandhttp://img.photobucket.com/albums/v102/mysticirishwolf/breastfeeding%20campaign/nipple-inhaler.jpg (accessed May 14, 2012).

42. For media coverage of the controversy, see Kaufman and Lee, "HHS Toned Down Breast-feeding Ads"; O'Mara, "Dastardly Deeds of the AAP."

43. Quoted from O'Mara, "Dastardly Deeds of the AAP."

44. Ibid.

45. "Ad Council Materials," Womenshealth.gov, http://www.womenshealth.gov/breastfeeding/government-in-action/national-breastfeeding-campaign/#materials (accessed May 9, 2012).

46. Orent, "The White House versus Mother's Milk."

47. American Academy of Family Physicians Breastfeeding Advisory Committee, "Breastfeeding, Family Physicians Supporting (Position Paper)," para. 8.

48. "The Cost of Not Breastfeeding," Florida Breastfeeding Coalition, Inc., http://www.flbreastfeeding.org/cost.htm (accessed May 9, 2012).

49. Hausman, *Viral Mothers*, 73.

50. Law, "Politics of Breastfeeding," 412.

51. Ibid.

52. Wolf, *Is Breast Best?*, 22.

53. Kukla, "Ethics and Ideology," 160.

54. Wolf, "What Feminists Can Do," 410.

55. Ibid.

56. Hausman, *Viral Mothers*, 72.

57. Rabin, "Vitamin D Deficiency."

58. Baker, Greer, and the Committee on Nutrition, "Clinical Report."

59. Schanler et al., "Concerns with Early Universal Iron Supplementation."

60. Ibid.

61. Hausman, *Viral Mothers*, 61–71.

62. Segal, *Health and the Rhetoric of Medicine*, 23.

63. Wolf, *Is Breast Best?*, xi, 16; see also Friedman, "For Whom is Breast Best?"; Knaak, "Deconstructing Discourse"; Law, "Politics of Breastfeeding."

64. Adams, Murphy, and Clarke, "Anticipation."

65. Miller, "Kairos in the Rhetoric of Science," 310.

Chapter Two: From "Wives' Tales and Folklore" to Scientific Fact

1. Hanson et al., "Antiviral and Antibacterial Factors in Human Milk," 141.

2. Gerrard, "Breast-Feeding," 757.

3. Tomasi, introduction, xiii.

4. AAP Work Group on Breastfeeding, "Breastfeeding," 1035.

5. AAP Section on Breastfeeding, "Breastfeeding," 496.

6. Haraway, "Biopolitics of Postmodern Bodies," 211.

7. Martin, *Flexible Bodies*, 36–37.

8. Ibid., 37.

9. Ibid.

10. Ibid., 119.

11. Rosenberg, *No Other Gods*.

12. Apple, *Mothers and Medicine*, 16–17; Wolf, *Don't Kill Your Baby*, 74–101.

13. Vahlquist, "Transfer of Antibodies," 305.

14. Martin, *Flexible Bodies*, 31.

15. Sabin, "Antipoliomyelitic Substance in Milk," 867.

16. Kirschner and Maguire, "Antileptospiral Effect of Milk," 564.

17. Györgi, "Hitherto Unrecognized Biochemical Difference," 98.

18. Baake, *Metaphor and Knowledge*, 114.

19. Journet, "Metaphor Ambiguity, and Motive in Evolutionary Biology," 411.

20. Keller, *Making Sense of Life*, 118.

21. The situation described here is one that Thomas S. Kuhn would describe as revolutionary science—science that is on the verge of a paradigm shift. There is definite overlap between Kuhn's concept of paradigm shift and the shift in metaphor that I discuss in this chapter. However, I have chosen to emphasize the metaphor concept rather than Kuhn's paradigm concept, because metaphor is most appropriate to a rhetorical understanding of the situation. (See Kuhn, *Structure of Scientific Revolution*.)

22. Vahlquist, "Transfer of Antibodies," 321.

23. Carter, "Stasis and Kairos," 99.

24. Prelli, *Rhetoric of Science*, 145.

25. Gage, "Adequate Epistemology for Composition," 167.

26. Hanson, "Comparative Immunological Studies."

27. Ibid., 262.

28. Mol, *Body Multiple*, 176.

29. Hanson and Johansson, "Immunological Characterization," 65.

30. Latour and Woolgar, *Laboratory Life*, 110. On the importance of images in establishing scientific and medical facts, see also Graham, "Agency and the Rhetoric of Medicine."

31. Martin, *Flexible Bodies*.

32. Kenny, Boesman, and Michaels, "Bacterial and Viral Coproantibodies." As evidence of its influence, this article currently has ninety-five citations, according to GoogleScholar, and it continues to be cited in recent years (the most recent citation at this time is a 2011 article).

33. Ibid., 202.

34. Ibid.

35. Ibid., 205.

36. Ibid., 209.

37. Winberg and Wessner, "Does Breast Milk Protect against Septicaemia?," 1094.

38. Ibid.

39. Ibid., 1091.

40. Ibid., 1094.

41. Hanson and Winberg, "Breast Milk and Defence against Infection," 845.

42. Ibid.

43. Ibid., 847.

44. Gerrard, "Breast-Feeding," 757.

45. Ibid., 763.

46. Ogra, Weintraub, and Ogra, "Immunologic Aspects of Human Colostrum and Milk," 247.

47. Ibid., 248.

48. Lemons, Stuart, and Lemons, "Breast-Feeding the Premature Infant," 112–13.

49. Ibid., 112.

50. Ibid., 113.

51. Ibid., 119.

52. Baake, *Metaphor and Knowledge*, 62.

53. Jerne, "Towards a Network Theory of the Immune System."

54. Tomasi, introduction, xiii.

55. Hanson et al., "Antiviral and Antibacterial Factors in Human Milk," 142.
56. Ibid.
57. Vahlquist, "Transfer of Antibodies," 318.
58. Newton and Newton, "Relation of the Let-Down Reflex," 726.
59. Ibid.
60. Egli, Egli, and Newton, "Influence of the Number of Breast Feedings," 314.
61. Schiebinger, *Nature's Body*, 53–54.
62. Martin, *Flexible Bodies*.
63. Starr, *Social Transformation*.
64. Martin, *Flexible Bodies*, 183.
65. Ibid.
66. See, for example, Blum, *At the Breast*; Carter, *Feminism, Breasts, and Breastfeeding*; Galtry, "Extending the Bright Line"; Hausman, *Mother's Milk*; Law, "Politics of Breastfeeding."
67. Friedman, "For Whom Is Breast Best?"; Knaak, "Deconstructing Discourse"; Kukla, "Ethics and Ideology"; Kukla, *Mass Hysteria*; Law, " Politics of Breastfeeding"; Wolf, *Is Breast Best?*
68. Martin, *Flexible Bodies*; Martin, "Woman in the Flexible Body"; Adkins, "Cultural Feminization."
69. AAP Task Force on Infant Feeding Practices, "Report of the Task Force."

Chapter Three: Articulating Knowledge and Practice

1. McCarthy and Gerring, "Revising Psychiatry's Charter Document"; Teston, "Grounded Investigation of Genred Guidelines."
2. Teston, "Grounded Investigation of Genred Guidelines," 323.
3. Althusser, *Humanist Controversy*; Gramsci, *Selection from the Prison Notebookss*; Grossberg, "Language and Theorizing in the Human Sciences"; Hall, "On Postmodernism."
4. Hall, "On Postmodernism," 141.
5. Ibid.
6. Slack, "Technical Communicator"; Slack, Miller, and Doak, "Technical Communicator."
7. Slack, Miller, and Doak, "Technical Communicator," 26.
8. Gerrard, "Breast-Feeding," 762.
9. AAP Nutrition Committee of the Canadian Paediatric Society and the Committee on Nutrition of the American Academy of Pediatrics, "Breast-Feeding," 597.
10. AAP Committee on Nutrition, "Encouraging Breast-Feeding," 658.
11. May, "'Infant Formula Controversy,'" 429.
12. AAP Task Force on the Promotion of Breast Feeding, "Promotion of Breastfeeding," 654.
13. Ibid., 655.
14. Ibid.
15. Ibid., 657.
16. Ibid., 658.
17. Ibid.
18. Ibid., 660.
19. Ibid., 661.
20. AAP Work Group on Breastfeeding, "Breastfeeding and the Use of Human Milk," 1035.
21. Ibid., 1036.

22. Ibid., 1035.

23. Slack, Miller, and Doak, "Technical Communicator," 27.

24. Gerrard, "Breast-Feeding"; AAP Nutrition Committee of the Canadian Paediatric Society and the Committee on Nutrition of the American Academy of Pediatrics, "Breast-Feeding"; AAP Committee on Nutrition, "Encouraging Breast-Feeding."

25. AAP Committee on Nutrition, "Nutrition and Lactation," 440.

26. Grant, "Letter to Ms. Lori Cooper."

27. Sanders, "Letter to Ms. Lori Cooper."

28. AAP Work Group on Breastfeeding, "Minutes," July 18, 1994.

29. Ibid.

30. AAP Work Group on Breastfeeding, "Intent for Statement."

31. AAP Work Group on Breastfeeding, "Intent for Subject Review."

32. On the role of policy documents in managing organizational uncertainty, see Bowker and Star, *Sorting Things Out*; McCarthy and Gerring, "Revising Psychiatry's Charter Document"; Sauer, *Rhetoric of Risk*.

33. AAP Work Group on Breastfeeding, "Breastfeeding and the Use of Human Milk," 1035.

34. Ibid.

35. AAP Task Force on Infant Feeding Practices, "Report of the Task Force."

36. Bauchner, Leventhal, and Shapiro, "Studies of Breast-Feeding and Infections."

37. Beaudry et al., "Relation between Infant Feeding and Infections"; Dewey et al., "Differences in Morbidity"; Duncan et al., "Exclusive Breast-Feeding."

38. AAP Work Group on Breastfeeding, "Breastfeeding and the Use of Human Milk," 1035.

39. Slack, Miller, and Doak, "Technical Communicator," 27.

40. Bowker and Star, *Sorting Things Out*, 82.

41. Slack, "Technical Communicator"; Slack, Miller, and Doak, "Technical Communicator."

42. Slack, Miller, and Doak, "Technical Communicator," 26.

43. See the appendix for more detailed information on the research participants quoted in this chapter. The names used are pseudonyms, and details about each participant are arranged in alphabetical order by pseudonym.

44. Slack, Miller, and Doak, "Technical Communicator," 28.

45. "Healthy People 2010," Office of Disease Prevention and Health Promotion, U.S. Department of Health and Human Services, http://www.healthypeople .gov/2010/?visit=1 (accessed May 8, 2012).

46. "National Breastfeeding Campaign," U.S. Department of Health and Human Services, http://www.womenshealth.gov/breastfeeding/programs/nbc/ (accessed May 8, 2012).

47. Bowker and Star, *Sorting Things Out*, 47–48.

48. AAP Task Force on Breastfeeding, "American Academy of Pediatrics Proposal"; see also "Breastfeeding Initiatives," American Academy of Pediatrics, http://www.aap .org/breastfeeding/sectionOnBreastfeeding.html (accessed May 10, 2012).

49. AAP Task Force on Breastfeeding, "American Academy of Pediatrics Proposal," 111.

50. AAP Work Group on Breastfeeding, "Minutes," December 5–6, 1998.

51. Ibid., February 27–28, 1999, 15.

52. Ibid., 16–17.

53. AAP Provisional Section on Breastfeeding, "Minutes," October 29–30, 2000.

54. AAP Section on Breastfeeding, "Breastfeeding and the Use of Human Milk," 496.

55. Ibid.
56. Ibid.
57. Ibid.
58. Ibid., 496–97.
59. Ibid., 497.
60. AAP Work Group on Breastfeeding, "Breastfeeding and the Use of Human Milk," 1037.
61. AAP Section on Breastfeeding, "Breastfeeding and the Use of Human Milk," 500.
62. Brockmann, *Exploding Steamboats*; Coogan, "Public Rhetoric and Public Safety"; Cook, "Writers and Their Maps"; Rude, "Toward an Expanded Concept of Rhetorical Delivery."
63. Rude, "Toward an Expanded Concept of Rhetorical Delivery," 272.
64. Ibid., 282.
65. Wright and Treacher, *Problem of Medical Knowledge*, 4.
66. Denny, "Evidence-Based Medicine."
67. Hall, "On Postmodernism," 141.

Chapter Four: Viral Rhetoric

1. "Breastfeeding: Baby's First Immunization," American Academy of Pediatrics, http://www.aap.org/breastfeeding/curriculum/documents/pdf/BFIZPoster.pdf (accessed May 10, 2012).
2. Lawrence and Pane, "Human Breast Milk"; Pabst et al., "Effect of Breast-Feeding on Immune Response."
3. "Dandelions," womenshealth.gov, http://www.womenshealth.gov/breastfeeding/government-in-action/national-breastfeeding-campaign/adcouncil/Dandelion.pdf (accessed May 10, 2012).
4. "Otoscopes," womenshealth.gov, http://www.womenshealth.gov/breastfeeding/government-in-action/national-breastfeeding-campaign/adcouncil/Otoscope_English.pdf (accessed May 10, 2012).
5. Video files and text transcripts of both commercials can be linked from womenshealth.gov, http://www.womenshealth.gov/breastfeeding/government-in-action/national-breastfeeding-campaign/#materials (accessed May 10, 2012).
6. "EarlyShield for Immune Support," Similac StrongMoms, http://similac.com/feeding-nutrition/baby-immune-system-prebiotics (accessed September 22, 2010).
7. "Enfamil Premium Infant," Enfamil, http://www.enfamil.com/app/iwp/enf10/content.do?dm=enf&id=-13538&iwpst=B2C&ls=0&csred=1&r=3462628889 (accessed May 10, 2012).
8. Edbauer, "Unframing Models of Public Distribution," 14.
9. Ibid., 18.
10. Bitzer, "Rhetorical Situation"; Vatz, "Myth of the Rhetorical Situation."
11. Biesecker, "Rethinking the Rhetorical Situation," 243.
12. Ibid., 112.
13. Edbauer, "Unframing Models of Public Distribution," 9.
14. Ibid., 13.
15. Ibid., 14.
16. On the importance of the immune system in current conceptions of health, see Haraway, "Biopolitics of Postmodern Bodies"; Martin, *Flexible Bodies*.
17. Lawrence and Pane, "Human Breast Milk."
18. Pabst et al., "Effect of Breast-Feeding on Immune Response."

19. See, for example, Fahnestock, "Accommodating Science "; Fahnestock, "Argument in Different Forums"; Fahenstock, *Rhetorical Figures in Science*; McDonald, "Language of Journalism"; Ryan, "Struggling to Survive"; Wilkes, "Public Dissemination of Medical Research."

20. "Science behind the Campaign—Campaign References," Womenshealth.gov, http://www.womenshealth.gov/breastfeeding/government-programs/national-breast feeding-campaign/index.cfm#c (accessed May 10, 2012).

21. "EarlyShield for Immune Support," Similac StrongMoms, http://similac.com/ feeding-nutrition/baby-immune-system-digestive-health (accessed May 10, 2012).

22. "Prebiotics," Similac StrongMoms, http://similac.com/baby-formula/digestive -health-prebiotics?autoplay=true (accessed September 22, 2010).

23. "Clinically Proven Triple Health Guard," Enfamil, http://www.enfamil.com/app/ iwp/enf10/content.do?dm=enf&id=-13538&iwpst=B2C&ls=o&csred=1&r= 3509379491 (accessed May 10, 2012).

24. Robert Krulwich, "Flu Attack! How a Virus Invades Your Body," National Public Radio, *Krulwich Wonders* (blog), October 23, 2009, http://www.npr.org/templates/ story/story.php?storyId=114075029

25. One of the difficult aspects of working with marketing websites such as those of formula manufacturers is that these sites are constantly changing. The language quoted here is no longer available at the site; it seems to have been replaced with language that says something similar but in simpler terms. For instance, there is no longer mention of the term *oligosaccharide*. All other quotations from Similac's and Enfamil's websites have been updated to reflect the sites' current language. However, in this instance, I felt it was important to keep in the language that I found in December 2009 because this language is central to the point I am discussing in this paragraph.

26. Lawrence and Pane, "Human Breast Milk," 8.

27. "Prebiotics," Similac StrongMoms, http://similac.com/feeding-nutrition/baby -immune-system-prebiotics (accessed December 30, 2009).

28. Lawrence and Pane, "Human Breast Milk," 8.

29. Fahnestock, "Accommodating Science."

30. Edbauer, "Unframing Models of Public Distribution," 14.

31. Yeutter, "Letter to the Honorable Tommy G. Thompson"; see also Kaufman and Lee, "HHS Toned Down Breastfeeding Ads."

32. "How is infant formula regulated in the United States?," U.S. Food & Drug Administration, http://www.fda.gov/Food/FoodSafety/Product-SpecificInformation/ InfantFormula/ConsumerInformationAboutInfantFormula/ucm108101.htm (accessed May 10, 2012).

33. "Dietary supplements," U.S. Food & Drug Administration, http://www.fda.gov/ Food/DietarySupplements/default.htm (accessed May 10, 2012).

34. "Overview of Dietary Supplements," U.S. Food and Drug Administration, http:// www.fda.gov/Food/DietarySupplements/ConsumerInformation/ucm110417.htm, para .3 (accessed May 10, 2012).

35. "GRAS Notification for Galacto-oligosaccharaides (GOS)," ENVIRON International Corporation, http://www.accessdata.fda.gov/scripts/fcn/gras_notices/grn000236 .pdf (accessed May 10, 2012).

36. Lawrence and Pane, "Human Breast Milk," 7.

37. WayBack Machine, accessed September 23, 2010, from http://www.archive.org/ index.php. If a user visits this URL and enters http://www.similac.com in the search box, a total of ninety-seven pages are returned, spanning the years 1998 to 2008. I examined all of these sites to determine the trends discussed in this paragraph.

38. "Similac Advance Infant Formula with Iron," Similac WelcomeAddition.com, November 2, 2005, accessed (using WayBack Machine) September 23, 2010, from http://web.archive.org/web/20051102092237/www.welcomeaddition.com/product1 .aspx.

39. U.S. General Accounting Office, *Breastfeeding*, 7.

40. Similar research strategies were used to explore the history of Enfamil's website. Using the WayBack Machine, http://www.enfamil.com was entered in the site's search engine. This search turns up a total of 475 pages, spanning 1998 to 2008. None of these archived sites mentions the Triple Health Guard additive, which leads me to surmise that this additive was first advertised sometime in 2009, which is when I began researching these sites.

41. See, for example, "Product Information," Mead-Johnson Nutritionals, January 25, 1999, accessed (through WayBack Machine) September 23, 2010, from http://web .archive.org/web/19990218064540/www.enfamil.com/products/index.html.

42. "Presentation on Breastfeeding Campaign with Campaign Research Findings," U.S. Department of Health and Human Services, http://www.womenshealth.gov/ breastfeeding/government-in-action/national-breastfeeding-campaign/#materials (accessed May 10, 2012).

43. "Concerns about Infant Formula Marketing and Additives," California WIC Association, http://www.calwic.org/storage/documents/federal/2010/formulabrief.pdf (accessed May 10, 2012).

44. On the medicalization of infant feeding, see Apple, *Mothers and Medicine*; Blum, *At the Breast*; Hausman, *Mother's Milk*.

45. See the appendix for more detailed information on each of the research participants quoted in this chapter. The names used are pseudonyms, and details about each participant are arranged in alphabetical order by pseudonym.

46. U.S. General Accounting Office, *Breastfeeding*, 7.

47. "Help Moms Beat the 'Booby Traps' with Best for Babes Ad Campaign," Best for Babes, http://www.bestforbabes.org/help-moms-beat-the-booby-traps/, para. 6 (accessed May 10, 2012).

48. "Born to Breastfeed: An Advertising Campaign Worth Watching," Kelly Burgess for iParenting, http://www.breastfeed.com/articles/breastfeeding-advocacy/born-to -breastfeed-2673/, para. 4 (accessed May 10, 2012).

Chapter Five: Rhetorical Agency and Resistance in the Context of Infant Feeding

1. Scott, Risky Rhetoric, 7.

2. Foucault, *Discipline and Punish*, 187.

3. Scott, *Risky Rhetoric*; Britt, *Conceiving Normalcy*; Lay, *Rhetoric of Midwifery*.

4. Foucault, *Discipline and Punish*, 27.

5. Graham, "Agency and the Rhetoric of Medicine"; Herndl, introduction; Hoover, "Rhetorical Agency"; Reeves, "Language, Rhetoric, and AIDS."

6. Reeves, "Language, Rhetoric, and AIDS," 153; Britt, *Conceiving Normalcy*, 147.

7. Britt, *Conceiving Normalcy*; Herndl, introduction; Herndl and Licona, "Shifting Agency"; Reeves, "Language, Rhetoric, and AIDS"; Schryer et al., "Structure and Agency"; Scott, *Risky Rhetoric*; Winsor, "Using Writing to Structure Agency."

8. Herndl and Licona, "Shifting Agency," 137.

9. Biesecker, "Michel Foucault and the Question of Rhetoric," 357.

10. Apple, *Mothers and Medicine*; Blum, *At the Breast*; Hausman, *Mother's Milk*; Maher, ed., *Anthropology of Breastfeeding*; Quandt, "Sociocultural Aspects of the

Lactation Process"; Van Esterik, "Politics of Breastfeeding"; Wolf, "What Feminists Can Do"; Yalom, *History of the Breast.*

11. AAP Work Group on Breastfeeding, "Breastfeeding and the Use of Human Milk," 1036.

12. Foucault, *Discipline and Punish.*

13. Cited in Biesecker, "Michel Foucault and the Question of Rhetoric," 355–56.

14. Ibid., 356.

15. AAP Work Group on Breastfeeding, "Breastfeeding and the Use of Human Milk," 1036.

16. Bourdieu, *Logic of Practice.*

17. Hale, *Medications and Mothers' Milk.*

18. "Hydrocodone," LactMed Drug and Lactation Database, http://toxnet.nlm.nih .gov/cgi-bin/sis/search/f?./temp/~zBsPb9:1 (accessed May 11, 2012).

19. AAP Section on Breastfeeding, "Breastfeeding and the Use of Human Milk," 497.

20. Ibid.

21. AAP Committee on Drugs, "Transfer of Drugs."

22. Lawrence and Lawrence, *Breastfeeding*, 66, 99–100.

23. Bailey, Pain, and Aarvold, "'Give It a Go' Breastfeeding Culture," 247.

24. Barton, "Infant Feeding Practices"; Lewallen et al., "Breastfeeding Support"; Mozingo et al., "'It Wasn't Working'"; Nelson, "Metasynthesis of Qualitative Breastfeeding Studies."

25. Bentley et al., "Infant Feeding Practices"; Cricco-Lizza, "Milk of Human Kindness"; Holmes et al., "Barrier to Exclusive Breastfeeding."

26. Although my research data focus on the United States, there is increasing evidence to suggest that many of these same anti-breastfeeding norms impact mothers' infant-feeding experiences in other countries as well, including developing nations where breastfeeding might have been traditionally perceived as the norm. One phenomenon that has received much attention from researchers interested in cross-cultural dimensions of infant feeding, for instance, is beliefs about insufficient milk as a justification for offering early supplementation or weaning. See, for example, Bezner Kerr et al., "'We Grandmothers Know Plenty'"; Caulfield, Huffman, and Piwoz, "Interventions to Improve"; Maher, *Anthropology of Breastfeeding.*

27. Bailey, Pain, and Aarvold, "'Give It a Go' Breastfeeding Culture"; Mozingo et al., "It Wasn't Working"; Nelson, "Metasynthesis of Qualitative Breastfeeding Studies."

28. Barton, "Infant Feeding Practices"; Lewallen et al., "Breastfeeding Support."

29. Blum, *At the Breast*; Wolf, "What Feminists Can Do"; Tavárez, "La Leche League."

30. Britt, *Conceiving Normalcy*, 13.

31. Ibid., 147.

32. Scott, *Risky Rhetoric*, 157.

33. Britt, *Conceiving Normalcy*, 147.

34. Ibid., 148.

35. Scott, *Risky Rhetoric*, 157.

36. Foucault, *History of Sexuality*, 95.

37. "Burger King: Breast-Feeding Fine," Arak, Joel, CBS News, Nov. 22, 2003, http:// www.cbsnews.com/stories/2003/11/22/national/main585110.shtml (accessed May 11, 2012).

38. angelawhit, "Applebee's Cooking Up Breastfeeding Trouble," *Blisstree Blog*, September 1, 2007, http://blisstree.com/live/applebees-cooking-up-breastfeeding-trouble/

?utm_source=blisstree&utm_medium=web&utm_campaign=b5hubs_migration (accessed May 11, 2012).

39. Certeau, *Practice of Everyday Life*, xxi.
40. Ibid.
41. Scott, *Risky Rhetoric*, 155.
42. Wolf, "Is Breast Really Best?," 596.

Chapter Six: Feminism, Rhetoric, and Breastfeeding

1. Westfall, "John McCain and Sarah Palin."
2. See, for example, McCarver, "Rhetoric of Choice."
3. Hausman, *Mother's Milk*, 193.
4. Ibid.
5. Blaney, "City Official Censors Art."
6. Bindley, "Breastfeeding Photos on Facebook Removed."
7. Hausman, *Viral Mothers*, 73.
8. Wolf, *Is Breast Best?*, 21.
9. Ibid., 72.
10. Ibid., 109.
11. Ibid.
12. See, for example, Kukla, "Ethics and Ideology."
13. Hopkinson, "Commentary," 637.
14. Ibid., 638.
15. Ibid., 645.
16. Heinig, "Burden of Proof," 374.
17. Wolf, *Is Breast Best?*, 1–12.
18. Ibid., 10–12.
19. Ibid., 37.
20. McKinney and Silver LLC, "National Breastfeeding Campaign."
21. Cricco-Lizza, "Infant-Feeding Beliefs"; Cricco-Lizza, "Milk of Human Kindness"; Guttman and Zimmerman, "Low-Income Mothers' Views"; Khoury et al., "Breast-Feeding Initiation"; Mozingo et al., "'It Wasn't Working.'"
22. Wolf, *Is Breast Best?*, 50.
23. Hopkinson, "Commentary," 647.
24. Emmons, *Black Dogs and Blue Words*, 7.
25. Walker, *Still Selling Out*.
26. Herndl, "Introduction."
27. Kukla, "Ethics and Ideology"; Kukla, *Mass Hysteria*; Law, "Politics of Breastfeeding"; Wolf, *Is Breast Best?*; Wolf, "Is Breast Really Best?"
28. Barton, "Design in Observational Research."
29. See, for example, Robin, *Bottle-Feeding without Guilt*, and the numerous sharply divided responses to that book, many of which are available online.

References

Adams, Vincanne, Michelle Murphy, and Adele E. Clarke. "Anticipation: Techno-science, Life, Affect, Temporality." *Subjectivity* 28 (2009): 246–65.

Adkins, Lisa. "Cultural Feminization: 'Money, Sex and Power' for Women." *Signs: Journal of Women in Culture and Society* 26 (2001): 669–95.

Althusser, Louis. *For Marx*. Translated by Ben Brewster. New York: Random House, 1970.

———. *The Humanist Controversy and Other Writings*. Translated by G. M. Goshgarian. London: Verso Books, 2003.

American Academy of Family Physicians Breastfeeding Advisory Committee. "Breastfeeding, Family Physicians Supporting (Position Paper)." http://www.aafp.org/online/en/home/policy/policies/b/breastfeedingpositionpaper.html (accessed May 7, 2012).

American Academy of Pediatrics Committee on Drugs. "The Transfer of Drugs and Other Chemicals into Human Milk." *Pediatrics* 108 (2001): 776–89.

American Academy of Pediatrics Committee on Fetus and Newborn. *AAP Standards and Recommendations for Hospital Care of Newborn Infants, Full-Term and Premature*. Evanston, Ill.: American Academy of Pediatrics, 1949.

American Academy of Pediatrics Committee on Nutrition. "Encouraging Breast-Feeding." *Pediatrics* 65 (1980): 657–58.

———. "Nutrition and Lactation." *Pediatrics* 68 (1981): 435–43.

American Academy of Pediatrics Nutrition Committee of the Canadian Paediatric Society and the Committee on Nutrition of the American Academy of Pediatrics. "Breast-Feeding: A Commentary in Celebration of the International Year of the Child." *Pediatrics* 62 (1978): 591–601.

American Academy of Pediatrics Provisional Section on Breastfeeding. "Minutes of the AAP Provisional Section on Breast-Feeding." October 29–30, 2000. (Available from Bakwin Library, 141 NW Point Boulevard, Elk Grove Village, Ill. 60007–1019.)

American Academy of Pediatrics Section on Breastfeeding. "Breastfeeding and the Use of Human Milk." *Pediatrics* 115 (2005): 496–506.

———. "Section on Breastfeeding." http://www.aap.org/breastfeeding/sectionOnBreastfeeding.html (accessed May 7, 2012).

American Academy of Pediatrics Task Force on Breastfeeding. "American Academy of Pediatrics Proposal for Establishment of a Provisional Section on Breastfeeding." October 7, 1999. (Available from Bakwin Library, 141 NW Point Boulevard, Elk Grove Village, Ill. 60007–1019.)

American Academy of Pediatrics Task Force on Infant Feeding Practices. "Report of the Task Force on the Assessment of the Scientific Evidence Relating to Infant-Feeding Practices and Infant Health." *Pediatrics* 74 Supplement (1984): 579–82.

American Academy of Pediatrics Task Force on the Promotion of Breast Feeding. "The Promotion of Breastfeeding." *Pediatrics* 69 (1982): 654–61.

American Academy of Pediatrics Work Group on Breastfeeding. "Breastfeeding and the Use of Human Milk." *Pediatrics* 100 (1997): 1035–39.

———. "Intent for Statement." September 20, 1994. (Available from Bakwin Library, 141 NW Point Boulevard, Elk Grove Village, Ill. 60007–1019.)

———. "Intent for Subject Review." September 20, 1994. (Available from Bakwin Library, 141 NW Point Boulevard, Elk Grove Village, Ill. 60007–1019.)

———. "Minutes of the AAP Work Group on Breast-Feeding." July 18, 1994. (Available from Bakwin Library, 141 NW Point Boulevard, Elk Grove Village, Ill. 60007–1019.)

———. "Minutes of the AAP Work Group on Breastfeeding." February 12, 1995. (Available from Bakwin Library, 141 NW Point Boulevard, Elk Grove Village, Ill. 60007–1019.)

———. "Minutes of the AAP Work Group on Breastfeeding." December 5–6, 1998. (Available from Bakwin Library, 141 NW Point Boulevard, Elk Grove Village, Ill. 60007–1019.)

———. "Minutes of the AAP Work Group on Breastfeeding." February 27–28, 1999. (Available from Bakwin Library, 141 NW Point Boulevard, Elk Grove Village, Ill. 60007–1019.)

Apple, Rima D. *Mothers and Medicine: A Social History of Infant Feeding, 1890–1950.* Madison: University of Wisconsin Press, 1987.

———. *Perfect Motherhood: Science and Childrearing in America.* New Brunswick, N.J.: Rutgers University Press, 2006.

Aristotle. *On Rhetoric: Theory of Civic Discourse.* Translated and edited by George A. Kennedy. New York: Oxford University Press, 1991.

Baake, Ken. *Metaphor and Knowledge: The Challenges of Writing Science.* Albany: State University of New York Press, 2003.

Bailey, Cathy, Rachel H. Pain, and Joan E. Aarvold. "A 'Give It a Go' Breastfeeding Culture and Early Cessation among Low-Income Mothers." *Midwifery* 20 (2004): 240–50.

Baker, Robert D., Frank R. Greer, and the Committee on Nutrition. "Clinical Report—Diagnosis and Prevention of Iron Deficiency and Iron-Deficiency Anemia in Infants and Young Children (0–3 Years of Age)." *Pediatrics* 126 (2010): 1040–50.

Bartlett, Alison. *Breastwork: Rethinking Breastfeeding.* Sydney: University of New South Wales Press, 2005.

Barton, Ellen. "Design in Observational Research on the Discourses of Medicine: Toward Disciplined Interdisciplinarity." *Journal of Business and Technical Communication* 15 (2001): 309–32.

Barton, Sharon J. "Infant Feeding Practices of Low-Income Rural Mothers." *American Journal of Maternal Child Nursing* 26 (2001): 93–97.

Bauchner, H., J. M. Leventhal, and E. D. Shapiro. "Studies of Breast-Feeding and Infections: How Good Is the Evidence?" *JAMA* 256 (1986): 887–92.

Baumslag, Naomi, and Dia L. Michels. *Milk, Money, and Madness: The Culture and Politics of Breastfeeding.* Westport, Conn.: Bergin & Garvey, 1995.

Beaudry, Micheline, Renee Dufour, and Sylvie Marcoux. "Relation between Infant Feeding and Infections during the First Six Months of Life." *Journal of Pediatrics* 126 (1995): 191–97.

Bentley, Margaret, et al. "Infant Feeding Practices of Low-Income, African-American, Adolescent Mothers: An Ecological, Multigenerational Perspective." *Social Science and Medicine* 49 (1999): 1085–1100.

Berg, Marc, and Annemarie Mol. *Differences in Medicine: Unraveling Practices, Techniques, and Bodies.* Durham: Duke University Press, 1998.

Berkenkotter, Carol. *Patient Tales: Case Histories and the Uses of Narrative in Psychiatry.* Columbia: University of South Carolina Press, 2008.

Bezner Kerr, Rachel, et al. "'We Grandmothers Know Plenty': Breastfeeding, Complementary Feeding, and the Multifaceted Role of Grandmothers in Malawi." *Social Science and Medicine* 66 (2008): 1095–1105.

Biesecker, Barbara. "Michel Foucault and the Question of Rhetoric." *Philosophy and Rhetoric* 25 (1992): 351–64.

———. "Rethinking the Rhetorical Situation from within the Thematic of Difference." *Philosophy and Rhetoric* 22 (1989): 110–29.

Bindley, Katherine. "Breastfeeding Photos on Facebook Removed from 'Respect the Breast' Page." *Huffpost Parents,* February 18, 2012. http://www.huffingtonpost .com/2012/02/18/breastfeeding-photos-facebook-respect-the-breast_n_1285264. html (accessed May 11, 2012).

Bitzer, Lloyd. "The Rhetorical Situation." *Philosophy and Rhetoric* 1 (1968): 1–15.

Blaney, Betsy. "City Official Censors Art for Display at Buddy Holly Center." *Lubbock Online-Lubbock Avalanche-Journal,* December 13, 2007. http://lubbockonline.com/ stories/121307/loc_121307034.shtml (accessed May 11, 2012).

Blum, Linda M. *At the Breast: Ideologies of Breastfeeding and Motherhood in the Contemporary United States.* Boston: Beacon Press, 1999.

Bourdieu, Pierre. *The Logic of Practice.* Translated by Richard Nice. Stanford: Stanford University Press, 1990.

Bowker, Geoffrey C., and Susan Leigh Star. *Sorting Things Out: Classification and Its Consequences.* Cambridge, Mass.: MIT Press, 1999.

Britt, Elizabeth C. *Conceiving Normalcy: Rhetoric, Law, and the Double Binds of Infertility.* Tuscaloosa: University of Alabama Press, 2001.

Brockmann, R. John. *Exploding Steamboats, Senate Debates, and Technical Reports: The Convergence of Technology, Politics and Rhetoric in the Steamboat Bill of 1838.* Amityville, N.Y.: Baywood Publishing Company, 2002.

Burgess, Kelly. "Born to Breastfeed: An Advertising Campaign Worth Watching." http:// www.breastfeed.com/articles/breastfeeding-advocacy/born-to-breastfeed-2673/ (accessed May 7, 2012).

Carter, Michael. "Stasis and Kairos: Principles of Social Construction in Classical Rhetoric." *Rhetoric Review* 7(1988): 97–112.

Carter, Pam. *Feminism, Breasts, and Breast-Feeding.* New York: St. Martin's, 1995.

Caulfield, Laura E., Sandra L. Huffman, and Ellen G. Piwoz. "Interventions to Improve Intake of Complementary Foods by Infants 6 to 12 Months of Age in Developing Countries: Impact on Growth and the Prevalence of Malnutrition and Potential Contribution to Child Survival." *Food and Nutrition Bulletin* 20, no. 2 (1999): 183–200.

Certeau, Michel de. *The Practice of Everyday Life.* Translated by Steven Rendall. Berkeley: University of California Press, 1984.

Clarke, Adele E., et al. "Biomedicalization: Techno-scientific Transformations of Health, Illness, and U.S. Biomedicine." *American Sociological Review* 68 (2003): 161–94.

Clifford, Steward H., et al. "Panel Discussion: A Program to Develop and Improve Facilities for the Care of Newborn Infants—Full Term and Premature," *Pediatrics* 2 (1948): 97–118.

Coogan, David. "Public Rhetoric and Public Safety at the Chicago Transit Authority: Three Approaches to Accident Analysis." *Journal of Business and Technical Communication* 16 (2002): 277–305.

Cook, Kelli Cargile. "Writers and Their Maps: The Construction of a GAO Report on Sexual Harassment." *Technical Communication Quarterly* 9 (2000): 53–76.

Creswell, John W. *Qualitative Inquiry and Research Design: Choosing among Five Approaches.* 2nd ed. Thousand Oaks, Calif.: Sage Publications, 2007.

Cricco-Lizza, Roberta. "Infant-Feeding Beliefs and Experiences of Black Women Enrolled in WIC in the New York Metropolitan Area." *Qualitative Health Research* 14 (2004): 1197–1210.

———. "The Milk of Human Kindness: Environmental and Human Interactions in a WIC Clinic That Influence Infant-Feeding Decisions of Black Women." *Qualitative Health Research* 15 (2005): 525–38.

Dancis, Joseph, John J. Osborn, and J. F. Julia. "Studies of the Immunology of the Newborn Infant: Effect of Dietary Protein on Antibody Production." *Pediatrics* 12 (1953): 395–99.

Denny, Keith. "Evidence-Based Medicine and Medical Authority." *Journal of Medical Humanities* 20 (1999): 247–63.

Dewey, Kathryn G., M. Jane Heinig, and Laurie A. Nommsen-Rivers. "Differences in Morbidity between Breast-Fed and Formula-Fed Infants." *Journal of Pediatrics* 126 (1995): 696–702.

Duncan, Burris, et al. "Exclusive Breast-Feeding for at Least 4 Months Protects against Otitis Media." *Pediatrics* 91 (1993): 867–72.

Edbauer, Jenny. "Unframing Models of Public Distribution: From Rhetorical Situation to Rhetorical Ecologies." *Rhetoric Society Quarterly* 35, no. 4 (2005): 5–24.

Egli, G. E., N. S. Egli, and Michael Newton. "The Influence of the Number of Breast Feedings on Milk Production." *Pediatrics* 27 (1961): 314–17.

Emmons, Kimberly K. *Black Dogs and Blue Words: Depression and Gender in the Age of Self-Care.* New Brunswick, N.J.: Rutgers University Press, 2010.

Fahnestock, Jeanne. "Accommodating Science: The Rhetorical Life of Scientific Facts." *Written Communication* 3 (1986): 275–96.

———. "Argument in Different Forums: The Bering Crossover Controversy." *Science, Technology, and Human Values* 14 (1989): 26–42.

———. *Rhetorical Figures in Science.* Oxford: Oxford University Press, 1999.

Foucault, Michel. *Discipline and Punish: The Birth of the Prison.* Translated by Alan Sheridan. New York: Vintage Books, 1977.

———. *The History of Sexuality: An Introduction, Volume 1.* Translated by Robert Hurley. New York: Vintage Books, 1978.

Friedman, May. "For Whom Is Breast Best? Thoughts on Breastfeeding, Feminism and Ambivalence." *Journal of the Association for Research on Mothering* 11, no. 1 (2009): 26–35.

Gage, John T. "An Adequate Epistemology for Composition: Classical and Modern Perspectives." In *Essays on Classical Rhetoric and Modern Discourse,* edited by Robert J. Connors, Lisa S. Ede, and Andrea A. Lunsford, 152–69. Carbondale: Southern Illinois University Press, 1984.

Galtry, Judith. "Extending the Bright Line: Feminism, Breastfeeding, and the Workplace in the United States." *Gender and Society* 14 (2000): 295–317.

Gerrard, John W. "Breast-Feeding: Second Thoughts." *Pediatrics* 54 (1974): 757–64.

Golden, Janet. *A Social History of Wet Nursing in America: From Breast to Bottle.* Cambridge: Cambridge University Press, 1996.

Graham, Scott S. "Agency and the Rhetoric of Medicine: Biomedical Brain Scans and the Ontology of Fibromyalgia." *Technical Communication Quarterly* 18 (2009): 376–404.

Gramsci, Antonio. *Selections from the Prison Notebooks.* Edited and translated by Q. Hoare and G. Nowell Smith. London: Lawrence and Wishart, 1971.

Grant, J. P. "Letter to Ms. Lori Cooper, Executive Director Healthy Mothers, Healthy Babies." January 27, 1994. (Available from Bakwin Library, 141 NW Point Boulevard, Elk Grove Village, Ill. 60007–1019.)

Grossberg, Lawrence. "Language and Theorizing in the Human Sciences." *Studies in Symbolic Interaction* 2 (1979): 189–231.

Guttman, Nurit, and Deena R. Zimmerman. "Low-Income Mothers' Views on Breastfeeding." *Social Science and Medicine* 50 (2000): 1457–73.

Györgi, Paul. "A Hitherto Unrecognized Biochemical Difference between Human Milk and Cow's Milk." *Pediatrics* 11 (1953): 98.

Hale, Thomas W. *Medications and Mothers' Milk: A Manual of Lactational Pharmacology*, 13th ed. Amarillo: Hale Publishing, 2008.

Hall, Stuart. "On Postmodernism and Articulation: An Interview with Stuart Hall." Edited by Lawrence Grossberg. *Journal of Communication Inquiry* 10, no. 2 (1986): 45–60.

Hanson, Lars A. "Comparative Immunological Studies of the Immune Globulins of Human Milk and of Blood Serum." *International Archives on Allergy* 18 (1961): 241–67.

Hanson, Lars A., et al. "Antiviral and Antibacterial Factors in Human Milk." In *Biology of Human Milk*, Nestle Nutrition Workshop Series, vol. 15, 141–57. New York: Raven Press, 1988.

Hanson, Lars A., and Bengt G. Johansson. "Immunological Characterization of Chromatographically Separated Protein Fractions from Human Colostrum." *International Archives on Allergy* 20 (1962): 65–79.

Hanson, Lars A., and Jan Winberg. "Breast Milk and Defence against Infection in the Newborn." *Archives of Disease in Childhood* 47 (1972): 845–48.

Haraway, Donna. "The Biopolitics of Postmodern Bodies: Constitutions of Self in Immune-System Discourse." In *Simians, Cyborgs, and Women: The Reinvention of Nature*, 203–30. New York: Routledge, 1991.

———. "Situated Knowledges: The Science Question in Feminism and the Privilege of Partial Perspective." In *Feminism/Science*, edited by Evelyn Fox Keller and Helen E. Longino, 249–63. Oxford: Oxford University Press, 1996.

Hausman, Bernice L. *Mother's Milk: Breastfeeding Controversies in American Culture.* New York: Routledge, 2003.

———. *Viral Mothers: Breastfeeding in the Age of HIV/AIDS.* Ann Arbor: University of Michigan Press, 2011.

Heinig, M. Jane. "The Burden of Proof: A Commentary on 'Is Breast Really Best': Risk and Total Motherhood in the National Breastfeeding Awareness Campaign." *Journal of Human Lactation* 23 (2007): 374–76.

Herndl, Carl. "Introduction to the Special Issue: The Legacy of Critique and the Promise of Practice." *Journal of Business and Technical Communication* 18 (2004): 3–8.

Herndl, Carl G., and Adele C. Licona. "Shifting Agency: Agency, *Kairos*, and the Possibilities of Social Action." In *Communicative Practices in Workplaces and the Professions*, edited by Mark Zachry and Charlatte Thralls, 133–53. Amityville, N.Y.: Baywood Publishing Company, 2007.

Holmes, Alison Vope, et al. "A Barrier to Exclusive Breastfeeding for WIC Enrollees: Limited Use of Exclusive Breastfeeding Food Package for Mothers." *Breastfeeding Medicine* 4 (2009): 25–30.

Hoover, Ryan S. "Rhetorical Agency, Social Structures, and Power Relations in the National Science Foundation's Grant Application Process." PhD diss., Texas Tech University, 2009.

Hopkinson, Judy M. "Commentary: Response to 'Is Breast Really Best? Risk and Total Motherhood in the National Breast-Feeding Awareness Campaign." *Journal of Health Politics, Policy, and Law* 32 (2007): 637–48.

Jerne, Neils K. "Towards a Network Theory of the Immune System." *Annales d' Immunologie* 125 (1974): 373–89.

Journet, Debra. "Metaphor, Ambiguity, and Motive in Evolutionary Biology: W.D. Hamilton and the 'Gene's Point of View.'" *Written Communication* 22 (2005): 379–420.

Kaufman, Marc, and Christopher Lee. "HHS Toned Down Breastfeeding Ads." *Washington Post*, August 31, 2007. http://www.washingtonpost.com/wp-dyn/content/article/2007/08/30/AR2007083002198.html (accessed May 8, 2012).

Keller, Evelyn Fox. *Making Sense of Life: Explaining Biological Development with Models, Metaphors, and Machines.* Cambridge: Harvard University Press, 2002.

Kenny, Jean F., Mary I. Boesman, and Richard H. Michaels. "Bacterial and Viral Copro-antibodies in Breast-Fed Infants." *Pediatrics* 39 (1967): 202–13.

Khoury, Amal J., et al. "Breast-Feeding Initiation in Low-Income Women: Role of Attitudes, Support, and Perceived Control." *Women's Health Issues* 15 (2005): 64–72.

Kirschner, L., and T. Maguire. "Antileptospiral Effect of Milk." *New Zealand Medical Journal* 54 (1955): 560–64.

Knaak, Stephanie. "Deconstructing Discourse: Breastfeeding, Intensive Mothering and the Moral Construction of Choice." In *Mother Knows Best: Talking Back to the "Experts,"* edited by Jessica Nathanson and Laura Camille Tuley, 79–90. Toronto: Demeter Press, 2008.

Koerber, Amy. "U.S. Breastfeeding Education and Promotion, 1978–99: A Feminist Rhetorical Analysis." PhD diss., University of Minnesota–Twin Cities, 2002.

———. "'You Just Don't See Enough Normal': Critical Perspectives on Infant-Feeding Discourse and Practice." *Journal of Business and Technical Communication* 19 (2005): 304–27.

Kuhn, Thomas S. *The Structure of Scientific Revolutions* 3rd ed. Chicago: University of Chicago Press, 1996.

Kukla, Rebecca. "Ethics and Ideology in Breastfeeding Advocacy Campaigns." *Hypatia* 21, no. 2 (2006): 157–80.

———. *Mass Hysteria: Medicine, Culture, and Mothers' Bodies.* Lanham, Md.: Rowman & Littlefield, 2005.

Latour, Bruno, and Steve Woolgar. *Laboratory Life: The Construction of Scientific Facts.* Princeton: Princeton University Press, 1986.

Law, Jules. "The Politics of Breastfeeding: Assessing Risk, Dividing Labor." *Signs: Journal of Women in Culture and Society* 25 (2000): 407–50.

Lawrence, Robert M., and Camille A. Pane. "Human Breast Milk: Current Concepts of Immunology and Infectious Diseases." *Current Problems in Pediatric Adolescent Health Care* 37 (2007): 7–36.

Lawrence, Ruth A., and Robert M. Lawrence. *Breastfeeding: A Guide for the Medical Profession.* 6th ed. Philadelphia: Elsevier Mosby, 2005.

Lay, Mary M. *The Rhetoric of Midwifery: Gender, Knowledge, and Power.* Piscataway, N.J.: Rutgers University Press, 2000.

Leach, Joan, and Deborah Dysart-Gale. "Why Ask Rhetorical Questions? Asking Rhetorical Questions of Health and Medicine." In *Rhetorical Questions of Health and Medicine*, edited by Joan Leach and Deborah Dysart-Gale, 1–8. Lanham, Md.: Lexington Books, 2011.

Lemons, P., Mary Stuart, and James A. Lemons. "Breast-Feeding the Premature Infant." *Clinics in Perinatology* 13 (1986): 111–22.

Lewallen, Lynn Porter, et al. "Breastfeeding Support and Early Cessation." *Journal of Obstetric, Gynecologic, & Neonatal Nursing* 35 (2006): 166–72.

Löwy, Ilana. *Between Bench and Bedside: Science, Healing, and Interleukin-2 in a Cancer Ward.* Cambridge: Harvard University Press, 1996.

Maher, Vanessa, ed. *The Anthropology of Breastfeeding: Natural Law or Social Construct.* Oxford: Berg, 1992.

Martin, Emily. *Flexible Bodies: Tracking Immunity in the American Culture—from the Days of Polio to the Age of AIDS.* Boston: Beacon Press, 1994.

———. "The Woman in the Flexible Body." In *Revisioning Women, Health, and Healing: Feminist, Cultural, and Technoscience Perspectives,* edited by Adele E. Clarke and Virginia L. Olesen, 97–115. New York: Routledge, 1999.

May, Charles D. "The 'Infant Formula Controversy': A Notorious Threat to Reason in Matters of Health." *Pediatrics* 68 (1981): 428–30.

McCarthy, Lucille P., and Joan Page Gerring. "Revising Psychiatry's Charter Document: DSM-IV." *Written Communication* 11 (1994): 147–92.

McCarver, Virgina. "The Rhetoric of Choice and Twenty-First-Century Feminism: Online Conversations about Work, Family, and Sarah Palin." *Women's Studies in Communication* 34 (2011): 20–41.

McDonald, Susan Peck. "The Language of Journalism in Hormone Replacement News." *Written Communication* 22 (2005): 275–97.

McKinney & Silver LLC, "National Breastfeeding Campaign Advertising Strategy" (Meeting minutes, January 3, 2003, archived at Bakwin Library, 141 NW Point Boulevard, Elk Grove Village, Ill. 60007–1019.)

Miller, Carolyn R. "The Aristotelian *Topos:* Hunting for Novelty." In *Rereading Aristotle's Rhetoric,* edited by Alan G. Gross and Arthur E. Walzer, 130–43. Carbondale: Southern Illinois University Press, 2000.

———. "Kairos in the Rhetoric of Science." In *A Rhetoric of Doing: Essays on Written Discourse in Honor of James L. Kinneavy,* edited by Stephen P. Witte and Neil Nakadate, 310–27. Carbondale: Southern Illinois University Press, 1992.

Mol, Annemarie. *The Body Multiple: Ontology in Medical Practice.* Durham: Duke University Press, 2002.

Mozingo, Johnie N., et al. "'It Wasn't Working.' Women's Experiences with Short-Term Breastfeeding." *MCN American Journal of Maternal Child Nursing* 25 (2000): 120–26.

Mykhalovskiy, Eric, Liza McCoy, and Michael Bresalier. "Compliance/Adherence, HIV, and the Critique of Medical Power." *Social Theory & Health* 2 (2004): 315–40.

Nelson, Antonia M. "A Metasynthesis of Qualitative Breastfeeding Studies." *Journal of Midwifery and Women's Health* 51 (2006): e13–20.

Newton, Niles Rumely, and Michael Newton. "Relation of the Let-Down Reflex to the Ability to Breast Feed." *Pediatrics* 5 (1950): 726–33.

Ogra, S. S., D. Weintraub, and P. L. Ogra. "Immunologic Aspects of Human Colostrum and Milk." *Journal of Immunology* 119 (1977): 245–48.

O'Mara, Peggy. "The Dastardly Deeds of the AAP." http://mothering.com/the-dastardly-deeds-of-the-aap (accessed May 8, 2012).

Orent, Wendy. "The White House versus Mother's Milk: The Bush Administration Squelched Ads Promoting the Benefits of Breast-Feeding." *Los Angeles Times,* September 30, 2007. http://www.latimes.com/news/opinion/la-op-orent30sep30,0,2428317.story (accessed May 8, 2012).

Pabst, Henry F., et al. "Effect of Breast-Feeding on Immune Response to BCG Vaccination." *Lancet* 333 (1989): 295–97.

Plato. *Gorgias.* In *The Rhetorical Tradition: Readings from Classical Times to the Present,* 2nd ed., edited by Patricia Bizzell and Bruce Herzberg, 80–138. Boston: Bedford / St. Martin's, 2001.

Popham, Susan L. "Forms as Boundary Genres in Medicine, Science, and Business." *Journal of Business and Technical Communication* 19 (2005): 279–303.

Powers, Grover F. "Some Observations on the Feeding of Premature Infants Based on Twenty Years' Experience at the New Haven Hospital." *Pediatrics* 1 (1948): 145–58.

Prelli, Lawrence J. *A Rhetoric of Science: Inventing Scientific Discourse.* Columbia: University of South Carolina Press, 1989.

Quandt, Sarah A. "Sociocultural Aspects of the Lactation Process." In *Breastfeeding: Biocultural Perspectives,* edited by Patricia Stuart-Macadam and Katherine A. Dettwyler, 127–44. New York: Aldine DeGruyter, 1995.

Rabin, Roni Caryn. "Vitamin D Deficiency May Lurk in Babies." *New York Times,* August 25, 2008. http://www.nytimes.com/2008/08/26/health/research/26rick.html (accessed May 10, 2012).

Ratcliffe, Krista. *Rhetorical Listening: Identification, Gender, Whiteness.* Carbondale: Southern Illinois University Press, 2005.

Reeves, Carol. "Establishing a Phenomenon: The Rhetoric of Early Medical Reports on AIDS." *Written Communication* 7 (1990): 393–416.

———. "Language, Rhetoric, and AIDS: The Attitudes and Strategies of Key AIDS Medical Scientists and Physicians." *Written Communication* 13 (1996): 130–57.

Robin, Peggy. *Bottle-Feeding without Guilt: A Reassuring Guide for Loving Parents.* Roseville, Ca.: Prima Publishing, 1995.

Rosenberg, Charles E. *No Other Gods: On Science and American Social Thought.* Baltimore: Johns Hopkins University Press, 1976.

Rude, Carolyn D. "Toward an Expanded Concept of Rhetorical Delivery: The Uses of Reports in Public Policy Debates." *Technical Communication Quarterly* 13 (2004): 271–88.

Ryan, Cynthia. "Struggling to Survive: A Study of Editorial Decision-Making Strategies at MAMM Magazine." *Journal of Business and Technical Communication* 19 (2005): 353–76.

Sabin, Albert B. "Antipoliomyelitic Substance in Milk of Human Beings and Certain Cows." *American Journal of Diseases in Children* 80 (1950): 866–67.

Sanders, Joe M. Letter to Ms. Lori Cooper, Executive Director Healthy Mothers, Healthy Babies Coalition, June 13, 1994. (Available from Bakwin Library, 141 NW Point Boulevard, Elk Grove Village, Ill. 60007-1019.)

Sauer, Beverly. *The Rhetoric of Risk: Technical Documentation in Hazardous Environments.* Mahwah, N.J.: Lawrence Erlbaum, 2003.

Sawicki, Jana. *Disciplining Foucault: Feminism, Power, and the Body.* New York: Routledge, 1991.

Schanler, Richard J., et al. "Concerns with Early Universal Iron Supplementation of Breastfeeding Infants" [E-letter]. *Pediatrics* 126 (October 28, 2010). http://pediatrics.aappublications.org/cgi/eletters/126/5/1040 (accessed May 10, 2012).

Schiebinger, Londa S. *Nature's Body: Gender in the Making of Modern Science.* Boston: Beacon Press, 1993.

Schryer, Catherine F., et al. "Structure and Agency in Medical Case Presentations." In *Writing Selves / Writing Societies,* edited by Charles Bazerman and David Russell, 62–96. WAC Clearinghouse, 2003. http://wac.colostate.edu/books/selves_societies/ (accessed May 8, 2012).

Scott, J. Blake. *Risky Rhetoric: AIDS and the Cultural Practices of HIV Testing.* Carbondale: Southern Illinois University Press, 2003.

Segal, Judy Z. *Health and the Rhetoric of Medicine.* Carbondale: Southern Illinois University Press, 2005.

———. "Writing and Medicine: Text and Context." In *Writing in the Workplace: New Research Perspectives,* edited by Rachel Spilka, 84–97. Carbondale: Southern Illinois University Press, 1993.

Selzer, Jack. "Rhetorical Analysis: Understanding How Texts Persuade Readers." In *What Writing Does and How It Does It,* edited by Charles Bazerman and Paul Prior, 279–308. Mahwah, N.J.: Lawrence Erlbaum, 2004.

Slack, Jennifer D. "The Technical Communicator as Author? A Critical Postscript." In *Issues of Power, Status and Legitimacy in Technical Communication: Evaluating the Social and Historical Process of Professionalization,* edited by Gerald Savage and Teresa Kynell, 193–207. Amityville, N.Y.: Baywood Publishing, 2003.

Slack, Jennifer D., David J. Miller, and Jeffrey Doak. "The Technical Communicator as Author: Meaning, Power, Authority." *Journal of Business and Technical Communication* 7 (1993): 12–36.

Spivak, Gayatri C. "More on Power/Knowledge." In *Rethinking Power,* edited by T. E. Wartenberg, 149–77. Albany, NY: SUNY Press, 1992.

Starr, Paul. *The Social Transformation of American Medicine.* New York: Basic Books, 1979.

Tavárez, Elizabeth W. "La Leche League International: Class, Guilt, and Modern Motherhood." *Proceedings of the New York State Communication Association* (2007): 1–12.

Teston, Christa B. "A Grounded Investigation of Genred Guidelines in Cancer Care Deliberations." *Written Communication* 26 (2009): 320–48.

Tomasi, Thomas B., Jr. "Introduction." In *Immunology of Breast Milk,* edited by Pearay L. Ogra and Delbert H. Dayton, xiii–xvi. New York: Raven Press, 1979.

U.S. General Accounting Office. *Breastfeeding: Some Strategies Used to Market Infant Formula May Discourage Breastfeeding; State Contracts Should Better Protect against Misuse of WIC Name.* Publication No. GAO-06-282. http://www.gao.gov/new.items/do6282.pdf (accessed May 8, 2012).

Vahlquist, Bo. "The Transfer of Antibodies from Mother to Offspring." *Advances in Pediatrics* 10 (1958): 305–38.

Van Esterik, Penny. "The Politics of Breastfeeding: An Advocacy Perspective." In *Breastfeeding: Biocultural Perspectives,* edited by Patricia Stuart-Macadam and Katherine A. Dettwyler, 145–66. Hawthorne, N.Y.: Aldine De Gruyter, 1995.

Vatz, Richard E. "The Myth of the Rhetorical Situation." *Philosophy and Rhetoric* 6 (1973): 154–61.

Walker, Marsha. *Still Selling Out Mothers and Babies: Marketing of Breast Milk Substitutes in the USA.* Weston, Mass.: NABA REAL, 2007.

Ward, Julie DeJager. *La Leche League: At the Crossroads of Medicine, Feminism, and Religion.* Chapel Hill: University of North Carolina Press, 2000.

Westfall, Sandra Sobieraj. "John McCain and Sarah Palin on Shattering the Glass Ceiling." *People,* August 29, 2008. http://www.people.com/people/article/0,,20222685,00.html (accessed May 8, 2012).

Wilkes, Michael S. "The Public Dissemination of Medical Research: Problems and Solutions." *Journal of Health Communication* 2 (1997): 3–15.

Winberg, Jan, and G. Wessner. "Does Breast Milk Protect against Septicaemia in the Newborn?" *Lancet* 297 (1971): 1091–94.

Winsor, Dorothy. "Using Writing to Structure Agency: An Examination of Engineers' Practice." *Technical Communication Quarterly* 15 (2006): 411–30.

Wolf, Jacqueline H. *Deliver Me from Pain: Anesthesia and Birth in America*. Baltimore: Johns Hopkins University Press, 2009.

——. *Don't Kill Your Baby: Public Health and the Decline of Breastfeeding in the Nineteenth and Twentieth Centuries*. Columbus: Ohio State University Press, 2001.

——. "What Feminists Can Do for Breastfeeding and What Breastfeeding Can Do for Feminists." *Signs: Journal of Women in Culture and Society* 31(2006): 397–424.

Wolf, Joan B. *Is Breast Best? Taking on the Breastfeeding Experts and the New High Stakes of Motherhood*. New York: New York University Press, 2011.

——. "Is Breast Really Best? Risk and Total Motherhood in the National Breastfeeding Awareness Campaign." *Journal of Health Politics, Policy, and Law* 32 (2007): 595–636.

Wright, Peter, and Andrew Treacher. *The Problem of Medical Knowledge: Examining the Social Construction of Medicine*. Edinburgh: Edinburgh University Press, 1982.

Yalom, Marilyn. *A History of the Breast*. New York: Alfred A. Knopf, 1997.

Yeutter, Clayton. "Letter to the Honorable Tommy G. Thompson, Secretary U.S. Department of Health and Human Services," February 17, 2004. http://media.washington post.com/wp-srv/health/documents/yeutterletters.pdf (accessed May 8, 2012).

Index

CPSIA information can be obtained at www.ICGtesting.com
Printed in the USA
LVOW11s0747090214

372803LV00005B/10/P

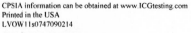